Current Cardiovascular Therapy

T0075719

Pablo Avanzas • Peter Clemmensen
Editors

Juan Carlos Kaski
Series Editor

Pharmacological Treatment of Acute Coronary Syndromes

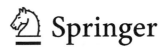 Springer

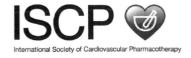 International Society of Cardiovascular Pharmacotherapy

Editors

Pablo Avanzas, MD, PhD, FESC
Department of Cardiology
Hospital Universitario
Central de Asturias
Oviedo
Spain

Peter Clemmensen, MD, PhD,
FESC
Department of Cardiology
The Heart Center
Rigshospitalet
University Hospital of
Copenhagen
Copenhagen
Denmark

ISBN 978-1-4471-5423-5   ISBN 978-1-4471-5424-2 (eBook)
DOI 10.1007/978-1-4471-5424-2
Springer London Heidelberg New York Dordrecht

Library of Congress Control Number: 2013950913

Printed on acid-free paper

Springer is part of Springer Science+Business Media (www.springer.com)

This book is dedicated to Prof. Juan Carlos Kaski,
President of ISCP

Series Preface

Cardiovascular pharmacotherapy is of fundamental importance for the successful management of patients with cardiovascular diseases. Appropriate therapeutic decisions require a proper understanding of the disease and a thorough knowledge of the pharmacological agents available for clinical use. The issue is complicated by the existence of large numbers of agents with subtle differences in their mode of action and efficacy and the existence of national and international guidelines, which sometimes fail to deliver a clear-cut message. Aggressive marketing techniques from pharma industry; financial issues at local, regional, or national levels; and time constraints make it difficult for the practitioner to – at times – be absolutely certain as to whether drug selection is absolutely appropriate. The International Society of Cardiovascular Pharmacotherapy (ISCP) aims at supporting evidence based, rational pharmacotherapy worldwide. This book series represents one of its vital educational tools. The books in this series aim at contributing independent, balanced, and sound information to help the busy practitioner to identify the appropriate pharmacological tools and to deliver rational therapies. Topics in the series include all major cardiovascular scenarios, and the books are edited and authored by experts in their fields. The books are intended for a wide range of healthcare professionals and particularly for younger consultants and physicians in training. All aspects of pharmacotherapy are tackled in the series in a concise and practical fashion. The books in this series provide a unique set of guidelines and examples that will prove valuable for patient management. They clearly articulate many of the dilemmas clinicians face when working to deliver sound therapies to their patients. The series will most certainly be a useful reference for those seeking to deliver evidence-based, practical, and successful cardiovascular pharmacotherapy.

Juan Carlos Kaski, DSc, DM (Hons),
MD, FRCP, FESC, FACC, FAHA
ISCP Current Cardiovascular Therapy Series

Preface

Acute coronary syndromes (ACS) require rapid intervention with pharmacologic therapies to treat and prevent coronary thromboembolism, and is essential to prepare the patient for revascularization procedures, especially percutaneous coronary intervention. The aims of treatment are to preserve patency of the coronary artery, augment blood flow through stenotic lesions, and reduce myocardial oxygen demand. Conventional treatment includes anti-ischemic, antiplatelet and anticoagulant therapy. All patients should receive antiplatelet agents, and patients with evidence of ongoing ischemia should receive aggressive medical intervention until signs of ischemia, as determined by symptoms and ECG, resolve. After a decade of relatively few advances in antithrombotic treatment, the clinical availability of potent new inhibitors of $P2Y_{12}$ platelet receptors has changed the ACS treatment paradigm. The most recent AMI – STEMI and NSTE-ACS guidelines of the European Society of Cardiology (ESC) have recommended ticagrelor and prasugrel in preference to clopidogrel for ACS patients, but globally clopidogrel is expected to remain a dominant therapy for the years to come. Furthermore, a group of novel oral anticoagulant and antiplatelet agents are promising for the acute management and secondary prevention in ACS. Triple therapy, while not initiated in the acute setting, may impact on future surgical and medical emergencies, and their management including bleeding complication should be known to health professionals across a wide spectrum of specialties. The ESC guidelines recommendations also differ for each of the antiplatelet and anticoagulant agent in terms of patient selection, pretreatment and timing of therapy; reflecting differences in the patient populations that were studied and the dissimilar safety profiles that emerged from trials. An unavoidable untoward consequence of increased antithrombotic effectiveness has been an increased risk, mostly in terms of bleeding.

The goal of this book is to update clinicians on the most recent data regarding the medical management of ACS patients. The authors have provided useful information and expert opinion that take into account results of large trials, European and American Guidelines, and real-life, day-to-day clinical practice.

Oviedo, Spain   Pablo Avanzas, MD, PhD, FESC
Copenhagen   Peter Clemmensen, MD, PhD, FESC
Denmark

Contents

Contributors

Dominick J. Angiolillo, MD, PhD Department of Cardiology, University of Florida College of Medicine-Jacksonville, Jacksonville, FL, USA

Pablo Avanzas, MD, PhD, FESC Department of Cardiology, Hospital Universitario Central de Asturias, Oviedo, Spain

Peter Clemmensen, MD, PhD, FESC Department of Cardiology, The Heart Center, Rigshospitalet, University Hospital of Copenhagen, Copenhagen, Denmark

Esteban López de Sá, MD, FESC Cardiology Department, Hospital Universitario La Paz, Instituto de Investigación La Paz IdiPaz, Madrid, Spain

Albert Ferro, BSc (Hons), MBBS, PhD, FRCP Department of Clinical Pharmacology, King's College London, London, UK

Francesco Franchi, MD Department of Cardiology, University of Florida College of Medicine-Jacksonville, Jacksonville, FL, USA

Gunnar Gislason, MD, PhD Department of Cardiology, Copenhagen University Hospital Gentofte, Hellerup, Denmark

Hyun-Jae Kang, MD, PhD Division of Cardiology, Duke Clinical Research Institute, Durham, NC, USA

Marcel Levi, MD, PhD Department of Medicine, Academic Medical Center, University of Amsterdam, Amsterdam, The Netherlands

Jose Lopez-Sendón, MD, PhD Cardiology Department, Hospital Universitario La Paz, Instituto de Investigación La Paz IdiPaz, Madrid, Spain

Cesar Morís, MD, PhD Department of Cardiology, Universidad de Oviedo, Oviedo, Spain

Ana Muñiz-Lozano, MD Department of Cardiology, University of Florida College of Medicine-Jacksonville, Jacksonville, FL, USA

Gabriella Passacquale, MD, PhD Department of Clinical Pharmacology, King's College London, London, UK

Matthew T. Roe, MD, MHS Division of Cardiology, Duke Clinical Research Institute, Durham, NC, USA

Fabiana Rollini, MD Department of Cardiology, University of Florida College of Medicine-Jacksonville, Jacksonville, FL, USA

Rikke Sørensen, MD, PhD Department of Cardiology, Copenhagen University Hospital Bispebjerg, København NV, Denmark

Abbreviations

ACS	Acute coronary syndrome
AF	Atrial fibrillation
APPRAISE-2	The Apixaban for Prevention of Acute Ischemic Events 2
ATLAS ACS 2-TIMI 51	The Anti-Xa Therapy to Lower Cardiovascular Events in Addition to Standard Therapy in Subjects with Acute Coronary Syndrome-Thrombolysis in Myocardial Infarction 51
ATRIA	Anticoagulation and Risk Factors in Atrial Fibrillation
BARC	Bleeding Academy Research Consort
CHA$_2$DS$_2$VASc	Congestive heart failure or left ventricular dysfunction hypertension, Age ≥75 (doubled), Diabetes, Stroke (doubled), Vascular disease, Age 65–74, Sex category (female)
CRUSADE	Can Rapid Risk Stratification of Unstable Angina Patients Suppress Adverse Outcomes with Early Implementation of ACC/AHA Guidelines
CURE	The Clopidogrel in Unstable Angina to Prevent Recurrent Events
GRACE	The Global Registry of Acute Coronary Events

HAS-BLED	Hypertension Abnormal Renal/Liver Function, Stroke, Bleeding History or Predisposition, Labile International Normalized Ratio, Elderly, Drugs/Alcohol
HEMORR(2)HAGES	Hepatic or Renal Disease Ethanol Abuse, Malignancy, Older Age, Reduced Platelet Count or Function, Re-Bleeding, Hypertension, Anemia, Genetic Factors, Excessive Fall Risk and Stroke
IHD	Ischemic heart disease
INR	International Normalized Ratio
MI	Myocardial infarction
NSTEMI	Non-ST-segment elevation myocardial infarction
PCI	Percutaneous coronary intervention
PLATO	The Study of Platelet inhibition and Patient Outcomes
PPI	Proton-pump inhibitors
RELY	The Randomized Evaluation of Long-Term Anticoagulation Therapy
STEMI	ST elevation myocardial infarction
TRITON-TIMI 38	Therapeutic Outcomes by Optimizing Platelet Inhibition with Prasugrel–Thrombolysis in Myocardial Infarction
UA	Unstable angina
WOEST	The What is the Optimal antiplatelet and anticoagulant therapy in patients with oral anticoagulation and coronary StenTing

Chapter 1
Anti-ischemic Therapy

Jose Lopez-Sendón and Esteban López de Sá

Introduction. Definition of Antiischemic Therapy

In a simple way, myocardial ischemia is secondary to a disbal-ance between oxygen supply in relation to the metabolic demands of the myocardium. Figure 1.1 depicts the principal components of this equation. In acute coronary syndromes plaque rupture and thrombosis play a major role, but other factors that decrease oxygen supply or increase myocardial metabolic demands contribute to ischemia and may be the principal cause of acute ischemia in absence of plaque rupture or coronary artery stenosis.

Reperfusion therapy constitutes the cornerstone for the modern treatment of patients with acute coronary syndromes. Before thrombolysis and percutaneous coronary revascularization, anti-ischemic therapy was the only effective treatment available and beta-blockers, nitrates and calcium channel blockers were routinely used in this clinical setting.

J. Lopez-Sendón, MD, PhD (✉) • E.L. de Sá, MD, FESC
Cardiology Department, Hospital Universitario La Paz,
Instituto de Investigación La Paz IdiPaz,
Paseo de la Castellana 261. Planta 1, Madrid 28046, Spain
e-mail: jlopezsendon@gmail.com

P. Avanzas, P. Clemmensen (eds.), *Pharmacological Treatment*
of Acute Coronary Syndromes, Current Cardiovascular Therapy,
DOI 10.1007/978-1-4471-5424-2_1,
© Springer-Verlag London 2014

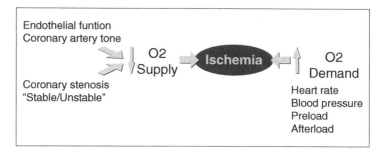

FIGURE 1.1 Myocardial ischemia is the result of multiple possible etiologies that may contribute to an imbalance in myocardial oxygen supply and demand

Today its role is less important; some of the classic drugs provide only a marginal benefit and new drugs with well demonstrated anti-ischemic efficacy in chronic treatments have been tested without much success during the first days of hours of acute coronary syndromes. Nevertheless, ischemia is frequent even after successful modern treatments [1] and anti-ischemic drugs are still needed, in particular for longer treatment strategies after the acute phase.

A significant number of compounds exert an anti-ischemic effect through various mechanism of action, including statins and antithrombotic drugs, but the term of anti-ischemic drugs is reserve for those with a direct anti-ischemic mechanism of action. Table 1.1 summarizes the different categories.

The content of this chapter is intended to provide the available information related to the clinical efficacy of anti-ischemic drugs early after acute coronary syndromes and its practical role in modern treatment strategies (Table 1.2).

Beta-Blockers

β-adrenergic antagonists (beta-blockers) bind selectively to the β-adrenoceptors producing a competitive and reversible antagonism of the effects of β-adrenergic stimuli on various organs. They play a crucial role in a broad spectrum

TABLE 1.1 Antiischemic drugs and principal mechanisms of action

Drug family	Mechanism of action	Anti-ischemic mechanism
Betablockers	Blockade of B receptors (competitive with chatecolamines)	Heart rate decrease
		Decrease contractility
		Afterload reduction
Nitrates	Nitric Oxide donor	Coronary artery vasodilation
		Preload reduction
Molsidomine	Nitric Oxide donor	Coronary artery vasodilation
		Preload reduction
Nicorandil	Potassium channel (KATP) opener	Free radical protection after reperfusion
	Nitrate-like effect	Nitrate-like effects
Calcium channel blockers	Blockade of voltage-gated calcium channels	Coronary and peripheral arterial vasodilation
	Decrease cellular Ca+ load	Decrease contractility
	Dihidropiridines nitric oxide donors	
Ranolazine	Late Na current blockade	Decreased ischemia induce by Ca+ overload secondary to ischemia
	Decrease cellular Ca+ load	
Ivabradine	If current blockade in sinus node	Pure reduction of heart rate
Trimetazidine	Metabolic	Reduction of free radicals
Other, no direct antiischemic effect	Statins	Endothelia function. Other pleiotropic effects
	Antithrombotics	Improve coronary flow

TABLE 1.2 Principal indications of anti-ischemic drugs in the early phase (first hours/days) of acute coronary syndromes

Drug family	Clinical settings	Precautions, contraindications
Betablockers oral	All cases w/o contraindications	Hypotension, heart failure, hemodynamic unstability, AV block, Asthma
Nitrates	Hypertension, ongoing non controlled ischemia, heart failure	Patients with hypotension
Molsidomine	Acute setting: None	
Calcium channel blockers	Acute setting: None	Hypotension, heart failure, hemodynamic unstability, AV block, heart failure
	Can be used later if myocardial ischemia, hypertension	
Ranolazine	Acute setting: None	
	Can be used later if myocardial ischemia	
Ivabradine	Acute setting: None	
	Can be used later if heart rate >60 beats/ minute	
Trimetazidine	Acute setting: None	

of cardiovascular diseases and have demonstrated clinical benefit in patients with unstable angina and acute myocardial infarction [2].

Mechanism of Action

The mechanisms of action of beta-blockers are diverse, not yet completely understood and probably with important differences between agents. The prevention of the cardiotoxic effects of catecholamines plays a central role [3]. Beta-blockers decrease myocardial oxygen demand by reducing heart rate, cardiac contractility, and systolic blood pressure [4]. These are the main anti-ischemic effects. In addition, prolongation of diastole caused by a reduction in heart rate may increase myocardial perfusion. Other beneficial actions include an antihypertensive effect associated with a decrease in cardiac output, inhibition of the release of renin and production of angiotensin II, blockade of presynaptic β2-adrenoceptors that increase the release of norepinephrine from sympathetic nerve terminals. Important in acute ischemia, beta-blockers exert a very effective antiarrhythmic action that may explain the reduction in cardiac death observed in patients of acute coronary syndromes and heart failure. Other more complex mechanisms probably are not relevant in the clinical setting of acute coronary syndromes.

Clinical Settings. Acute Myocardial Infarction

Beta-blockers limit infarct size, reduce life-threatening arrhythmias, relieve pain and reduce mortality including sudden death [2, 5–11]. Two large trials were particularly relevant to guide the use of beta-blockers during the first hours of AMI. In the First International Study of Infarct Survival (ISIS-1) trial [8] patients within 12 h of evolution were randomised to receive iv atenolol followed by oral administration for 7 days, or conventional treatment, revealing a significant reduction in mortality at 7 days (3.7 % vs 4.6 %; equivalent to 6 lives saved per 1,000 treated) (Fig. 1.2). The benefit was mainly due to a reduction in heart rupture and was evident by the end of day 1 and sustained at 1 month and 1 year. In the other large study, the Metoprolol in Myocardial Infarction (MIAMI) [9], iv metoprolol followed by oral administration did not significantly reduce 15-day mortality as compared to placebo (4.3–4.9 % (ns)). A metaanalysis of 28 early trials of iv beta-blockers [11] revealed an absolute reduction of short-term mortality from 4.3 to 3.7 % (7 lives saved/1,000 patients treated). This significant albeit small benefit was demonstrated before the reperfusion era. Similar

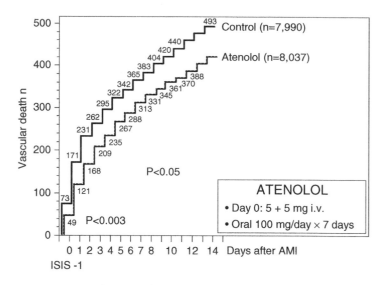

FIGURE 1.2 Cumulative vascular mortality in the groups of patients allocated to atenolol and placebo in the ISIS-1 trial (Reprinted with permission from ISIS-1 (First International Study of Infarct Survival) Collaborative Group [8])

findings were reported in a more recent metaanalysis of 52 trials, most of them including a small number of patients [12].

Three trials of randomised iv beta-blockade were conducted after the widespread use of reperfusion therapy in AMI [13–15], but the number of events was too small to establish clear conclusions. In the second Thrombolysis in Myocardial Infarction (TIMI-II) trial [13], thrombolysed patients were randomly assigned to early iv and oral metoprolol versus oral administration after day 6. Reinfarction and recurrent ischaemia were less frequent in the early beta-blocker group and when treatment was administered within 2 h of symptom onset, there was a reduction of the composite endpoint of death or reinfarction.

The COMMIT trial [15] Metoprolol (15 mg iv, then 200 mg oral daily) 45,000 Chinese patients with suspected acute STEMI within 24 h of evolution were randomly assigned to metoprolol (15 mg iv, then 200 mg oral daily) or placebo. About half received thrombolytic therapy. Exclusion criteria were shock at admission, systolic blood pressure <100 mmHg, heart rate <50 bpm and AV block. Mean treatment and follow up was 16 days. The study failed to demonstrate a reduction of total mortality in patients receiving metoprolol (Fig. 1.3), the benefit of metoprolol was limited to a reduction in arrhythmic dead (1.7 % vs 2.2 %; p < 0.01) and re-infarction (2 % vs 2.5 %; p < 0.002), somehow counterbalanced by an increase in mortality secondary to cardiogenic shock. The overall effect on death, reinfarction, cardiac arrest, or shock was significantly adverse during days 0–1 and significantly beneficial thereafter. There was substantial net hazard in haemodynamically unstable patients, and moderate net benefit in those who were relatively stable. The results of this somehow polemic trial, strongly suggest that intravenous beta-blockers should not be routinely used in patients with acute myocardial infarction in particular if the present heart failure or hemodynamic instability.

A global metaanalysis including these modern trials still provide evidence for benefit (Fig. 1.4), although some restrictions have to be considered and the metaanalysis includes completely different trials belonging to different times [15].

Registries offer a practical insight for the use of beta-blockers in the reperfusion era. Data from the US National Registry of Myocardial Infarction 2 [16] showed that immediate beta-blocker administration in patients with AMI treated with t-PA reduces the occurrence of intracranial haemorrhage, although this benefit is small (0.7 % and 1.0 %; 3 patients/1,000 treated). However, a post-hoc analysis of the first Global utilization of streptokinase and t-PA for occluded coronary arteries (GUSTO-I) trial and a systematic review of the available experience do not support the routine, early, *intravenous* use of beta-blockers [17, 18], at least when thrombolytic treatment or primary percutaneous intervention is performed. New data from the PAMI (Primary Angioplasty in AMI) Stent-PAMI, Air-PAMI and CADILLAC (Controlled Abciximab and Device

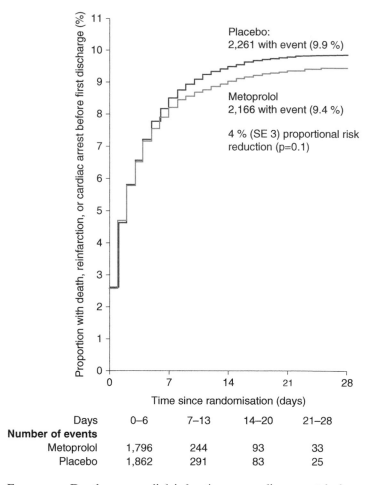

FIGURE 1.3 Death, myocardial infarction or cardiac arrest before hospital discharge in the COMMIT trial. No statistical differences were observed between metoprolol and placebo (Reprinted with permission from COMMIT (ClOpidogrel and Metoprolol in Myocardial Infarction Trial) Collaborative Group [15])

Investigation to Lower Late Angioplasty Complications) trials seem to demonstrate a reduction in mortality when beta-blockers are used before primary percutaneous interventions [19–21].

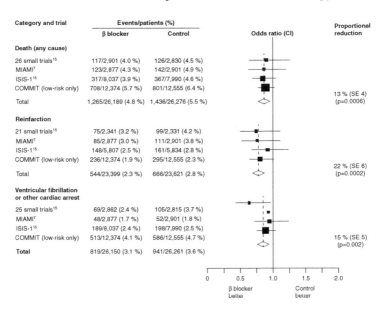

FIGURE 1.4 Metaanalysis of betablockers in patients with acute myocardial infarction, demonstrating a benefit in outcomes: mortality, myocardial infarction and ventricular fibrillation or other cardiac arrest (Reprinted with permission from COMMIT (ClOpidogrel and Metoprolol in Myocardial Infarction Trial) Collaborative Group [15])

In 13,110 patients with STEMI who received beta-blockers during the index hospitalization in the GRACE registry (emery) intravenous beta-blocker use (adjusted odds ratio 1.46, 95 % CI 1.31–1.64, P≤0.0001) and delayed beta-blocker use (after 1st 24 h) (adjusted odds ratio 1.35, 95 % CI 1.19–1.54, P≤0.0001) were associated with a higher composite outcome of death, cardiogenic shock, sustained ventricular fibrillation/ventricular tachycardia, and new heart failure when compared to early (1st 24 h) oral beta-blocker use. There was a reduction in mortality in patients who had delayed beta-blocker administration (adjusted odds ratio 0.56, 95 % CI 0.41–0.78, P ≤ 0.001) [22].

This data suggests that in acute STEMI early intravenous beta-blockers and delayed beta-blockers were associated with worse short-term outcomes compared with early oral administration.

Non ST Segment Elevation Acute Coronary Syndromes

There are few randomised studies with beta-blockers in patients with unstable angina and non Q wave myocardial infarction [23–25], and the new non-ST elevation ACS terminology makes the analysis of possible effect even more difficult. Henceforth, the recommendations are based on small studies in unstable angina as well as in the evidence in acute ST elevation myocardial infarction and stable patients with ischaemia and previous myocardial infarction. In fact, there are few studies in patients with unstable angina comparing beta-blockers with placebo A meta-analysis suggested that beta-blocker treatment was associated with a 13 % relative reduction in risk of progression to AMI [26]. A retrospective analysis from the Cooperative Cardiovascular Project [27] indicates that the relative risk of death was lower in patients with non Q wave myocardial infarction receiving beta-blockers. Pooled data from 2,894 patients with acute coronary syndromes included in five randomized, controlled trials of abciximab during coronary intervention showed a reduction of 30 day and 60 day mortality associated with the use of beta-blockers [28]. There is no evidence that any specific beta-blocking agent is more effective in producing beneficial effects in unstable angina and oral therapy should be aimed to achieving a target heart rate between 50 and 60 beats per minute.

In a cohort of 7,106 patients with NSTEMI from the GRACE registry [29], beta-blocker therapy was initiated within the first 24 h in 76 % of patients with NSTEMI (79 % with Killip class I vs 62 % with class II/III; p < 0.001). Failure to initiate beta-blockers within the first 24 h was associated with lower rates of subsequent beta-blocker therapy and other evidence-based therapies. Early beta-blocker therapy was correlated with lower hospital mortality for NSTEMI patients (OR 0.58, 95 % CI 0.42–0.81) and for those with Killip class II/III (OR 0.39, 95 % CI 0.23–0.68) with a trend toward lower mortality in the Killip class I group

(OR 0.77, 95 % CI 0.49–1.21). At 6 months post discharge, early BB use was associated with lower mortality in NSTEMI patients (OR 0.75, 95 % CI 0.56–0.997) with a trend toward lower mortality in patients with Killip class I or II/III.

Beta-blockers can increase coronary artery tone and are contraindicated in vasospastic angina without obstructive lesions [30].

Adverse Events

In general, β-adrenergic inhibitors are well tolerated, but serious side-effects may occur, especially when these agents are used in large doses [2]. Beta-blockers reduce heart rate and may cause extremebradycardia and AV block. Beta-blockers can also increase the coronary vasomotor tone, in part because of unopposed α-adrenergic mediated vasoconstriction. Beta-blockers can lead to a life-threatening increase in airway resistance and are contraindicated in patients with asthmaor bronchospastic chronic obstructive pulmonary disease. In some patients with chronic obstructive pulmonary disease, the potential benefit of using beta-blockers may outweigh the risk of worsening pulmonary function.

Contraindications

The contraindications to initiate beta-blocker treatment include asthma, symptomatic hypotension or bradycardia and severe decompensated heart failure. Contraindications may be relative, in patients in whom the benefit of therapy may outweigh the risk of untoward effects. Chronic obstructive lung disease without bronchospastic activity and peripheral vascular disease are not considered as absolute contraindications and high risk patients may obtain a significant benefit from this therapy [27, 28]. Diabetes or intermittent lower limb claudication are not absolute contraindications for beta-blockers use [2]. Heart failure during the acute setting of myocardial infarction is a formal contraindication for the use of intravenous beta-blockers. However, oral beta-blockers can be safely administered in patients with heart failure when the patient is stable and without need of intravenous inotropic support [31].

Drug Interactions

Beta-blockers may show pharmacokinetic and pharmacodynamic interactions with other drugs [2]. Aluminium salts, cholestyramine, and colestipol may decrease the absorption of beta-blockers. Alcohol, phenytoin, rifampicin, and phenobarbital, as well as smoking, induce hepatic biotransformation enzymes and decrease plasma concentrations and elimination half-lives of lypophilic beta-blockers. Cimetidine and hydralazine may increase the bioavailability of propranolol and metoprolol by reducing hepatic blood flow. Caution should be exercised in patients who are taking verapamil, diltiazem or various antiarrhythmic agents, which may depress sinus-node function or AV conduction. Additive effects on blood pressure between beta-blockers antagonists and other antihypertensive agents are often observed. Indometacin and other nonsteroidal anti-inflammatory drugs antagonize the antihypertensive effects of beta-blockers.

Dosing of Beta-Blockers

Appropriate dosing of beta-blockers varies with the clinical characteristics of the patient and the selected beta-blocker. Atenolol, metoprolol and carvedilol are the beta-blockers with the largest experience in the setting of acute coronary syndromes.

Calcium Channel Blockers

Calcium Channel Blockers (CHB) exert an anti-ischaemic effect through several mechanisms. The reduce afterload as the decrease blood pressure and contractility, have a vasodilatory effect in the coronary arteries and non-hydrop-iridines reduce heart rate [32]. Clinical trials with verapamil, diltiazem and nifedipine failed to demonstrate a consistent significant benefit in patients with acute coronary syndromes in studies conducted in the early 1980s with low use of antiaggregants, beta-blockers, statins, and revascularization. In the DAVIT-1 trial, treatment was started with 0.1 mg/kg verapamil i.v. and 120 mg/day orally on admission followed by 120 mg three times daily, or matched placebo. Mortality and reinfarction rates were similar in both groups of treatment during hospitalization and after 6 and 12-month follow-up of continuous treatment [33] (Fig. 1.5). In the Multicenter Diltiazem Reinfarction Study, conducted in 576 patients recovering from acute non-Q-wave MI treated with either diltiazem or placebo, treatment was initiated 24–72 h after the onset of MI and continued for 14 days. Active treatment did not modify total mortality, but reduced the early reinfarction rate compared with placebo (9.3 % vs 5.2 %, P < 0.03) [34].

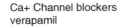

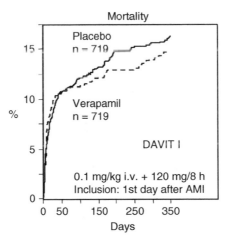

FIGURE 1.5 Mortality rate was similar in the groups treated with verapamil and placebo in the DAVIT-1 trial in patients with acute myocardial infarction (Reprinted with permission from The Danish Study Group on Verapamil in Myocardial Infarction [33])

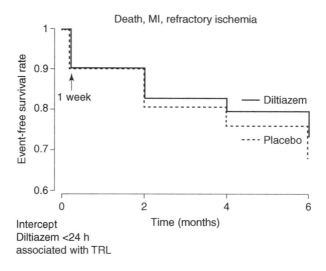

FIGURE 1.6 Mortality, myocardial infarction and refractory ischemia in the INTERCEPT trial, comparing diltiacem against placebo in patients with acute myocardial infarction (Reprinted with permission from Boden et al. [35])

In another prospective, randomized, double-blind, sequential trial in 874 patients with acute myocardial infarction, but without congestive heart failure, who first received thrombolytic agents (INTERCEPT trial), patients received either oral diltiazem or placebo, initiated within 36–96 h of infarct onset, and given for up to 6 months. Diltiazem did not reduce the cumulative occurrence of cardiac death, nonfatal reinfarction, or refractory ischemia during a 6-month follow-up (Fig. 1.6), but the need for revascularization was lower in the diltiazem group [35]. There is no information related to the possible benefit of CCB in patients with ACS treated according to contemporary strategies.

Hydropiridines have been also tested in acute coronary syndromes, and no benefit could be demonstrated in any of the trials. The NAMIS study [36] found that in patients with ischemic pain of >45 min duration nifedipine therapy (20 mg orally every 4 h for 14 days) did not prevent progression of threatened myocardial infarction to the acute event or limit infarct size in patients who experienced infarction. Among the 171 patients randomly assigned to drug or placebo, 6 months mortality did not differ between both groups (8.5 % for placebo vs 10.1 % for nifedipine), but mortality in the 2 weeks after randomization was significantly higher for nifedipine-treated patients (0 % for placebo vs 7 % for nifedipine, P = 0.018). The results indicate that nifedipine did not reduce the likelihood of progression from threatened myocardial infarction (TMI) to acute MI. In addition, nifedipine did not limit infarct size in those patients with TMI in whom infarction evolved or in patients in whom infarction was already in progress at the time of randomization. The reason for the lack of beneficial effect may have been the detrimental effects of the reduction in coronary blood flow caused by nifedipine-induced hypotension that may outweighed the beneficial effects of a decrease in afterload produced by the drug.

Accordingly, there is no evidence to recommend the routine use of calcium channel blockers as anti-ischemic therapy in patients with acute coronary syndromes.

Nitrates

Nitrates have been the all-time anti-ischemic agents in patients with acute coronary syndromes, chronic angina and secondary prevention. They quickly relieve acute episodes of angina and sublingual administration of short acting nitrates have been and still are the recommended medication to jugulate acute episodes of angina. In a small percentage of patients, nitroglycerin can open an otherwise occluded coronary artery during an episode of chest pain (Fig. 1.7).

Nitrates produce nonspecific smooth muscle relaxation through direct tissue action. This effect is independent of any known neurotransmitter [37]. At the level of the smooth muscle fiber, nitrates facilitate formation of nitric oxide (NO) that stimulates guanalyl cyclase activity, and increases the intracellular concentration of cGMP. CGMP decreases the

16   J. Lopez-Sendón and E.L. de Sá

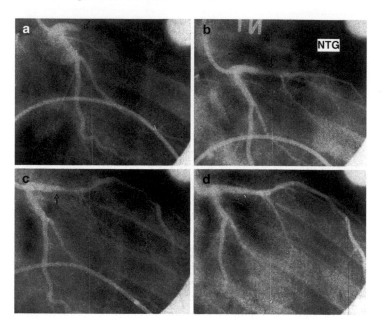

FIGURE 1.7 Coronary angiography in a patient with acute myo-cardial infarction. (**a**) Complete proximal occlusion of the left anterior descending coronary artery. (**b**) Restoration of flow after administration of nitroglycerine. (**c, d**) Final results after coronary angioplasty

intracellular concentration of free calcium, thereby causing smooth-muscle relaxation. Nitrates may combine with endogenous sulfhydryl groups, forming S-nitrositols (R-SNO) that subsequently converts to NO. Under physiologic conditions, the endothelium releases NO that acts as an endogenous nitrate, producing coronary vasodilation. In patients with ischemic heart disease, in whom the coronary endothelium is damaged, nitrates induce the formation of NO in smooth muscle cells, producing vasodilatation. Nitrates, present tachyfilaxia, and its effect disappears with time [38].

The primary action of nitrates is vasodilation, which is attributable primarily to nitrate-induced relaxation of vascular smooth muscle in veins, arteries, and arterioles. The metabolic conversion of organic nitrates to nitric oxide (NO) at or near the plasma membrane of the vascular smooth muscle cell represents the cellular basis for the vasodilatory action of these compounds. Believed to be an endothelium-derived relaxing factor (EDRF), NO is an important endogenous modulator of vascular tone. Nitrate administration has been viewed as a means of providing an exogenous source of NO that may help replenish or restore the actions of EDRF, which are usually impaired in patients with coronary artery atherosclerosis.

The reduction in right and left ventricular preload resulting from peripheral vasodilation, particularly in the splanchnic and mesenteric circulations, combined with afterload reduction resulting from arterial vasodilation, decreases cardiac work and lowers myocardial oxygen requirements. As a consequence, the ratio of myocardial oxygen demand to myocardial oxygen supply improves, and myocardial ischemia is alleviated. Because of their hemodynamic profile, nitrates are particularly useful in patients with impaired LV systolic function or heart failure. Additionally, both direct vasodilator effect of nitrates on the coronary bed and drug-induced prevention of episodic coronary artery vasoconstriction can increase global and regional myocardial blood flow, improving the subendocardial-epicardial blood flow ratio. Enlargement of obstructive atherosclerotic lesions containing intact vascular smooth muscle can increase the caliber of some stenoses, improving coronary flow. Nitrates also have been shown to dilate coronary collateral vessels, reverse vasoconstriction of small coronary arteries distal to a coronary obstruction, and reduce platelet aggregation.

Clinical Benefit

Few earlier trials prospectively randomized patients with acute coronary syndromes to explore the clinical efficacy of nitrates and most information is focusing on infarct size, enzymatic release and other surrogates for clinical efficacy; besides, the number of patients we were very small to draw conclusions.

In one of such trials, Judgutt et al. [39] 310 patients were randomly allocated to i.v. niroglycerin and control groups. Nitroglycerin infusion was titrated to lower mean blood pressure by 10 % in normotensive and 30 % in hypertensive patients, but not below 80 mmHg, and was maintained for 39 h.

Compared with controls, nitroglycerin decreased creatine kinase infarct size. Other indexes of infarct size (i.e. left ventricular asynergy, left ventricular ejection fraction, and Killip class score) also improved. Infarct-related major complications were less frequent in the NG than the control groups: infarct expansion syndrome, left ventricular thrombi thrombus, cardiogenic shock and infarct extension. Mortality was less in NG than in control groups in-hospital (14 % vs 26 %, $p < 0.01$), at 3 months (16 % vs 28 %, $p < 0.025$) and 12 months (21 % vs 31 %, $p < 0.05$), but this advantage was only found in patients with anterior Q wave infarction. Greater benefit on infarct size occurs with early timing (<4 h) and target mean blood pressure ≥ 80 mmHg.

These fantastic results prompted the organization of several megatrials in order to ascertain that nitrates should be routinely used in all patients with acute coronary syndromes. None demonstrated any relevant clinical benefit.

The GISSI-3 study was a multicentre randomized clinical trial to assess the efficacy of lisinopril, transdermal glyceryl trinitrate, and their combination in improving survival and ventricular function after acute myocardial infarction [40]. The GISSI-3 trial randomly assigned 19,394 patients within 24 h of symptom onset to a 24-h infusion of nitroglycerin (beginning within 24 h of onset of pain), followed by topical nitroglycerin (10 mg daily) for 6 week (with patch removed at bedtime, allowing a 10-h nitrate-free interval to avoid tolerance), or control. Approximately 50 % of patients in the control group received nitrates on the first day or two at the discretion of their physician, a major mistake in the design of the trial. There was an insignificant, and certainly non clinical relevant, reduction in mortality at 6 weeks in the group randomly assigned to nitrate therapy alone, compared with the control group (6.52 % vs 6.92 %, respectively) (Fig. 1.8).

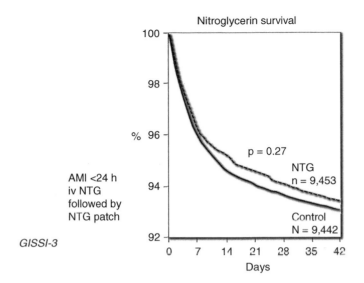

FIGURE 1.8 Survival curves in patients with acute myocardial infarction treated with nitroglycerine or placebo in the GISSI-3 trial (Reprinted with permission from Gruppo Italiano per lo Studio della Sopravvivenza nell'infarto Miocardico [40])

There were no significant differences between nitroglycerin-allocated and control patients in rates of reinfarction, revascularization procedures, persistent hypotension or renal dysfunction. The nitrate group had a lower rate of reinfarction angina (P = 0.03) and cardiogenic shock (P = 0.009). However, there was a significant excess of stroke rate in the nitrate group compared with controls (P = 0.027).

Another megatrial was organized to demonstrate that 5-isosorbide mononitrate, and oral nitrate with somehow a prolonged action for several hours. The purpose of the ISIS 4 study [41] was the reliable assessment of the effects on mortality and major morbidity of the addition of three widely used treatments in patients with definite or suspected acute myocardial infarction. 58,050 patients were randomized in a "2 × 2 × 2 factorial" design. The treatment comparisons were: (1) 1 month of oral captopril versus matching placebo; (2) 1

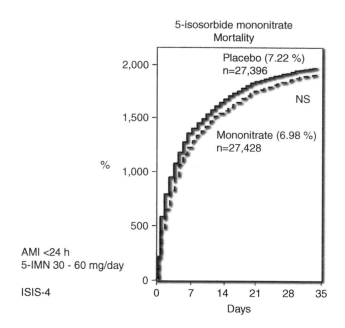

FIGURE 1.9 Mortality in patients with acute myocardial infarction treated with 5-isosorbide monotitrate or placebo in the ISIS 4 trial (Reprinted with permission from ISIS-4 (Fourth International Study of Infarct Survival) Collaborative Group [41])

month of oral controlled-release mononitrate (30 mg initial dose titrated up to 60 mg once daily) versus matching placebo, and (3) 24 h intravenous magnesium sulphate versus open control. Patients entering in the study up to 24 h (median 8 h) after the onset of suspected acute MI. At 5-weeks follow-up, there were 2,129 (7.34 %) deaths recordedamong 29,018 mononitrate-allocated patients compared with 2,190 (7.54 %) among 29,032 patients allocated matching placebo (P = 0.3) (Fig. 1.9). Follow-up to 1 year did not indicate any further divergence or convergence of the survival curves following 1 month of oral mononitrate. There were not differences in the incidence of reinfarction, post infarction angina or heart failure, but severe hypotension requiring termination of study treatment was more frequent in the nitrate group (8.1 % mononitrate vs 6.7 % placebo,

P < 0.0001). The high number of patent included in the trial permitted to explore different subgroups, but the study was consistently neutral in all.

A meta-analysis including the GISSI 3 and ISIS 4 data in addition of 20 small trial (11 by intravenous and by 9 oral administration) involving over 81,000 patients indicates that the role of nitrates in the treatment of acute coronary syndromes is marginal [41] and its use should be restricted to control hypertension, pulmonary congestion or refractory ischemia.

Molsidomine

In the believe that nitric oxide donors were potentially highly beneficial to control acute or chronic ischemia, other compounds were investigated in this clinical settings. In the ESPRIM trial, molsidomine, with and active metabolite, linsidomine, a nitric oxide donor was compared with placebo in a large-scale trial including 4,017 patients with acute myocardial infarction. Patients without signs of overt heart failure (Killip III/IV) were randomly assigned in a double-blind design within 24 h of symptom onset to receive molsidomine 1 mg/h intravenously for 48 h, followed by 16 mg molsidomine by mouth daily for 12 days, or an identical placebo [42]. The molsidomine and placebo groups showed similar all-cause 35-day mortality (8.4 % vs 8.8 %, p = 0.66), Similarly, no differences were found for long-term mortality (mean follow-up 13 months; 14.7 % vs 14.2 %, p = 0.67) (Fig. 1.10). The two groups showed similar frequencies of major and minor adverse events; only headache was significantly more common in the molsidomine group. It is still not clear whether nitric oxide donors can improve survival in higher-risk myocardial infarction patients.

Nicorandil

Adenosine triphosphate sensitive potassium channel openers (KATP) exert cardioprotectiveeffects in ischemic myocardium mimicking ischemic preconditioning. Nicorandil is

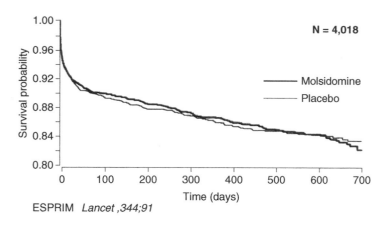

FIGURE I.10 Survival curves for patients allocated to molsidomine or placebo in the ESPRIM trial (Reprinted with permission from European Study of Prevention of Infarct with Molsidomine (ESPRIM) Group [42])

a KATP channel opener with additional properties similar to those of nitrate nitrates [43]. Several studies have been conducted in patients with acute myocardial infarction with and without reperfusion, trying to demonstrate some protective effect of nicorandil. The largest study, the J-MIND [44] included 545 patients with acute infarction undergoing reperfusion and failed to demonstrate benefit on the primary endpoint (infarct size measured by creatin kinase levels and Leith ventricular function evaluated with ventricular agiography).

In a meta-analysis of 17 studies including over 1,500 patients [45] nicorandil treatment reduced the incidence of TIMI flow grade ≤ 2 in the culprit artery, was associated with greater LVEF than placebo and no beneficial effect was observed on the peak creatine kinase value.

In conclusion, nicorandil treatment adjunctive to reperfusion therapy has some beneficial effects on microvascular function and on functional recovery after AMI but there is no clinical evidence of benefit and hence no indication in acute coronary syndromes.

Ranolazine

Ranolazine, a piperazine derivative, selectively inhibits the late inward sodium current (late I_{Na}) [46], a pathological current which occurs in ischemic conditions. Blocking late I_{Na} attenuates ischemia related myocardial sodium overload and, subsequently, intracellular calcium overload, a mediator of further myocardial ischemia. It is thought that the reduction in diastolic calcium overload improves myocardial relaxation and reduces left ventricular diastolic stiffness, which in turn may enhance myocardial perfusion and reduce subendocardial oxygen demand. Ranolazine produces anti-ischemic effects without depressing hemodynamic function while exerting minimal effects on heart rate and blood pressure. Ranolazine is approved for the treatment of chronic angina.

The MERLIN trial was designed to explore the efficacy of ranolazine against placebo in patients with acute coronary syndromes. The trial included 6,560 patients within 48 h of ischemic symptoms [47]. Ranolazine was initiated intravenously and followed by oral ranolazine extended-release 1,000 mg twice daily, or matching placebo. The primary efficacy end point was a composite of cardiovascular death, myocardial infarction, or recurrent ischemia through the end of study. And was not significantly different in the ranolazine and placebo groups (21.8 % vs 23.5 %, p=0.11). Recurrent ischemia was reduced in the ranolazine group (13.9 %) vs 16.1 %, p<0.03 and in patients with chronic angina reduced the composite outcome of cardiovascular death and myocardial infarction [48]. The trial concluded that the effect was not enough to recommend ranolazine in acute coronary syndromes but the trial provided support for the safety and efficacy of ranolazine to treat chronic stable angina.

Trimetazidine

Trimetazidine is an antianginal agent that has no negative inotropic or vasodilator properties. Although it is thought to have direct cytoprotective actions on the myocardium, the mechanisms by which this occurs are not completely defined but probably it shifts cardiac energy metabolism from fatty acid oxidation to glucose oxidation by inhibiting mitochondrial enzymes [49].

The EMIP–FR (European Myocardial Infarction Project – Free Radicals) was a prospective, double-blind, European multicentre trial compare the effect of trimetazidine versus placebo administered to 19,725 patients during the acute phase of myocardial infarction (within the first 24 h) on long and short-term mortality [50]. Stratification was according to thrombolytic therapy (56 %) or not (44 %). An intravenous bolus injection of trimetazidine (40 mg) was given just before or simultaneously with thrombolysis, followed by continuous infusion (60 mg/24 h) for 48 h. Overall, no difference was found between trimetazidine and placebo for the main end-point, short-term (35-day) mortality, (P = 0.98) in an intention-to-treat analysis. This was the result of opposing trends in the two strata. Thrombolysed patients showed a tendency towards more short-term deaths with trimetazidine, compared to placebo (11.3 %, vs 10.5 %, p = 0.15) and non thrombolysed patients the converse (trimetazidine: 14.0 %, placebo: 15.1 %, p = 0.14). For non thrombolysed patients, in a per-protocol analysis the beneficial effect of trimetazidine became statistically significant (trimetazidine: 13.3 %, placebo: 15.1 %, P = 0.027).

In conclusion, trimetazidine does not reduce mortality in patients undergoing thrombolytic therapy; however, it might have some beneficial effect fornon thrombolysed patients.

If Channel Blockers. Ivabradine

Heart rate plays a major role in some major factors related with the pathophysiology of ACS. Increased heart rate is associated with endothelial dysfunction, plaque instability and ruptureand a decreased threshold for ventricular fibrillation. A high heart rate in patients with ACS increases cardiac work and myocardial oxygen consumption, and reduces diastolic myocardial perfusion time. This can produce an imbalance between myocardial oxygen demand and supply, contributing to ischemia in patients with ACS [51]. In addition, after an acute complete coronary artery occlusion, collateral circulation plays a crucial role and is related to prognosis and collaterals are much more frequently visible on angiography in presence lower hear rates.

In the contemporary Global Registry of Acute Coronary Events (GRACE), including patients with ST-elevation myocardial infarction (STEMI), non-STEMI, and unstable angina, heart rate was an independent prognostic factor in an elaborated model, with an attributable risk for in-hospital and post-discharge mortality of 5–10 % for each 10 bpm increase in heart rate [52]. Similar findings were observed in other trials and registries [53]. Despite of this evidence, A relatively recent observational study demonstrated that only a minority of post-ACS patients (5.3 %) treated according to current guidelines reached the recommended level of heart rate during their hospital stay [54].

Some of the benefit obtained with beta-blockers in patients with ACS may be derived from a reduction in heart rate, with a direct relationship between the obtained heart rate reduction and the reduction in infarct size, reinfarction, and clinical outcomes including mortality [55]. This relationship has not been demonstrated with calcium channel blockers.

Ivabradine, the only available selective inhibitor of the I_f current, reduces heart rate without affecting cardiac contractility or blood pressure. In experimental models, ivabradine reduced oxygen consumption, increased myocardial blood flow, improved endothelial and myocardial function, and reduced infarct size [55].

In the VIV*If*Y trial intravenous ivabradine reduce heart rate and left ventricular volume as compared with placebo in patients with STEMI and primary PCI. This pilot trial showed that the use of the drug was safe and opens an opportunity to explore a new family drugs for the treatment of ischemia in patients with acute coronary syndromes.

Conclusions

Anti-ischemic agents still play a role in acute coronary syndromes in the reperfusion era. However, only betablockers can be recommended as a routine treatment in absence of contraindications. Beta-blockers should be started *per os* as soon as possible and its intravenous administration should be reserved for special cases such as patients with severe arrhythmias. Other antiischemic therapies should only be considered in special situations and for the treatment of myocardial ischemia after the acute episode.

References

1. Arnold SV, Morrow D, Ley Y, Cohen DL, Mahoney EM, Braunwald E, Cahn PS. Economic impact of angina after an acute coronary syndrome: insights from the MERLIN-TIMI 36 trial. Circ Cardiovasc Qual Outcomes. 2009;2:344–53.
2. López-Sendón J, Swedberg K, McMurray J, Tamargo J, Maggioni AP, Dargie H, Tendera M, Waagstein F, Kiekshus J, Lechat P, Torp-Pedersen C. Expert consensus document on angiotensin converting enzyme inhibitors in cardiovascular disease. The task Force on ACE-inhibitors of the European Society of Cardiology. Eur Heart J. 2004;25:1454–70.
3. Waagstein F. Beta-blockers in congestive heart failure: the evolution of a new treatment concept-mechanism of action and clinical implications. J Clin Basic Cardiol. 2002;5:215–23.
4. Frishman WH. Multifactorial actions of beta-adrenergic-blocking drugs in ischemic heart disease: current concepts. Circulation. 1983;67(Suppl I):I-11–8.
5. Hjalmarson Å, Elmfeldt D, Herlitz J, et al. Effect on mortality of metoprolol in acute myocardial infarction. A double-blind randomised trial. Lancet. 1981;ii:823–7.
6. Richterova A, Herlitz J, Holmberg S, et al. The göteborg metoprolol trial in acute myocardial infaction. Effects on chest pain. Am J Cardiol. 1984;53:32D–6.
7. Norris RM, Brown MA, Clarke ED, et al. Prevention of ventricular fibrillation during acute myocardial infarction by intravenous propranolol. Lancet. 1984;2:883–6.
8. ISIS-1 (First International Study of Infarct Survival) Collaborative Group. Randomised trial of intravenous atenolol among 16027 cases of suspected acute myocardial infarction: ISIS-1. Lancet. 1986;II:57–66.
9. The MIAMI Trial Research Group: Metoprolol in acute myocardial infarction (MIAMI). Am J Cardiol. 1985;56:1G–57.

10. Ryden L, Ariniego R, Arnman K, et al. A double-blind trial of meto-prolol in acute myocardial infarction. Effects on ventricular tachyarrhythmias. N Engl J Med. 1983;308:614–8.
11. Yusuf S, Lessem J, Pet J, et al. Primary and secondary prevention of myocardial infarction and strokes. An update of randomly allocated controlled trials. J Hypertens. 1993;11 Suppl 4:S61–73.
12. Freemantle N, Cleland J, Young P, et al. Beta blockade after myocardial infarction. Systematic review and meta regression analysis. BMJ. 1999;318:1730–7.
13. Roberts R, Rogers WJ, Mueller HS, et al. Immediate versus deferred beta-blockade following thrombolytic therapy in patients with acute myocardial infarction (TIMI) IIB study. Circulation. 1991;83:422–37.
14. Van de Werf F, Janssens L, Brzostek T, et al. Short term effect of early intravenous treatment with beta-adrenergic blocking agents or a specific bradycardia agent in patients with acute myocardial infarction receiving thrombolytic therapy. J Am Coll Cardiol. 1993;2:407–16.
15. COMMIT (ClOpidogrel and Metoprolol in Myocardial Infarction Trial) Collaborative Group. Early intravenous then oral metoprolol in 45,852 patients with acute myocardial infarction: randomised placebo controlled trial. Lancet. 2005;366:1622–32.
16. Barron HV, Rundle AC, Gore JM, et al., for the Participants in the national registry of myocardial infarction-2. Intracranial hemorrhage rates and effect of immediate beta-blocker use in patients with acute myocardial infarction treated with tissue plasminogen activator. Am J Cardiol. 2000;85:294–8.
17. Pfisterer M, Cox JL, Granger CG, et al. Atenolol use and clinical outcomes after thrombolysis for acute myocardial infarction. The GUSTO-I experience. Global utilization of streptokinase and tPA (alteplase) for occluded coronary arteries. J Am Coll Cardiol. 1998;32:634–40.
18. The Task Force on the management of ST-segment elevation acute myocardial infarction of the European Society of Cardiology (ESC). ESC guidelines for the management of acutemyocardial infarction in patients presenting with ST-segment elevation. Eur Heart J. 2012;33:2569–619.
19. Harjai KJ, Stone GW, Boura J, et al. Effects of prior beta-blocker therapy on clinical outcomes after primary coronary angioplasty for acute myocardial infarction. Am J Cardiol. 2003;91:655–60.
20. Halkin A, Nikolsky E, Aymong E, et al. The survival benefit of periprocedural beta-blockers in patients with acute myocardial infarction undergoing primary angioplasty is determined by use of these drugs before admission. Am J Cardiol. 2003;92(Suppl L):228L.
21. Kernis SJ, Arguya KJ, Boura J, et al. Does beta-bloquer therapy improbé clinical outcomes of acute myocardial infarction after successful primary angioplasty? A pooled análisis from the primary angioplasti in myocardial infarction-2 (PAMI-2), No surgery on-site

(noSOS), stetn PAMI and Air PAMI trials. Circulation. 2003;108(Suppl IV):416–7.

22. Scheuble A, Emery M, López-Sendón J, de Lopez Sa E, Fondard O, Dabbous OH, Eagle KA, Anderson FA, Steg PG. Patterns of early use of intravenous and oral beta-blockers in ST-segment elevation myocardial infarction in the reperfusion era. The Global Registry of Acute Coronary Events. Eur Heart J. 2005;26(Abstract Suppl):159.

23. Gottlieb S, Weisfeldt ML, Ouyang P, et al. Effect of the addition of propranolol to therapy with nifedipine for unstable angina pectoris: a randomized, double-blind, placebo-controlled trial. Circulation. 1986;3:331–7.

24. Telford A, Wilson C. Trial of heparin versus atenolol in prevention of myocardial infarction in intermediate coronary syndrome. Lancet. 1981;1:1225–8.

25. Lubsen JTJ. Effcacy of nifedipine and metoprolol in the early treatment of unstable angina in the coronary care unit: findings from the Holland Interuniversity Nifedipine/metoprolol Trial (HINT). Am J Cardiol. 1987;60:18A–25.

26. Yusuf S, Witte J, Friedman L. Overview of results of randomized trials in heart disease: unstable angina, heart failure, primary prevention with aspirin and risk factor modifications. JAMA. 1988;260:2259–63.

27. Gottlieb S, McCarter R, Vogel R. Effect of beta-blockade on mortality among high risk patients after myocardial infarction. N Engl J Med. 1998;338:489–97.

28. Ellis K, Tcheng JE, Sapp S, Topol EJ, Lincoff AM. Mortality benefit of beta blockade in patients with acute coronary syndromes undergoing coronary intervention: pooled results from the Epic, Epilog, Epistent, Capture and Rapport Trials. J Interv Cardiol. 2003;16:299–305.

29. Emery M, López-Sendón J, Steg PG, Anderson Jr FA, Dabbous OH, Scheuble A, Eagle KA. Patterns of use and potential impact of early beta-blocker therapy in non-ST-elevation myocardial infarction with and without heart failure: the Global Registry of Acute Coronary Events. Am Heart J. 2006;152:1015–21.

30. Tilmant PY, Lablanche JM, Thieuleux FA, et al. Detrimental effect of propranolol in patients with coronary arterial spasm countered by combination with diltiazem. Am J Cardiol. 1983;52:230–3.

31. Members of the CAPRICORN Steering Committee on behalf of the investigators and committees. CAPRICORN. Effect of carvedilol on outcome after myocardial infarction in patients with left ventricular dysfunction. Lancet. 2001;357:1385–90.

32. Church J, Zsotér T. Calcium antagonistic drugs. Mechanism of action. Can J Physiol Pharmacol. 1980;58:254–64.

33. The Danish Study Group on Verapamil in Myocardial Infarction. Verapamil in acute myocardial infarction. Eur Heart J. 1984;5;516–28.

34. Gibson RS, Boden WE, Theroux P, Strauss HD, Pratt CM, Gheorghiad M, Capone RJ, Crawford MH, Schlant RC, Kleiger RE. Diltiazem and reinfarction in patients with non-Q-wave myocardial infarction. Results of a double-blind, randomized, multicenter trial. N Engl J Med. 1986;315:423.

35. Boden W, Gilst W, Scheldewaert R, Starkey S, Carlier M, Julian D, Whitehead A, Bertrand M, Col J, Pedersen O, Lie K, Santoni JP, Fox KM and for the Incomplete Infarction Trial of European Research Collaborators Evaluating Prognosis post-Thrombolysis (INTERCEPT). Diltiazem in acute myocardial infarction treated with thrombolytic agents: a randomised placebo controlled trial. Lancet. 2000;355:1751–6.

36. Muller JE, Morrison J, Stone PH, Rude RE, Rosner B, Roberts R, Pearle DL, Turi ZG, Schneider AD, Serfas DH. Nifedipine therapy for patients with threatened and acute myocardial infarction: a randomized, double-blind, placebo-controlled comparison. Circulation. 1984;69:740–7.

37. Torfgård KE, Ahlner J. Mechanisms of action of nitrates. Cardiovasc Drugs Ther. 1994;8:701–17.

38. Klemenska E, Beresewicz A. Bioactivation of organic nitrates and the mechanism of nitrate tolerance. Cardiol J. 2009;16:11–9.

39. Jugdutt BI, Warnica JW. Intravenous nitroglycerin therapy to limit myocardial infarct size, expansion, and complications. Effect of timing, dosage, and infarct location. Circulation. 1988;78:906–19.

40. Gruppo Italiano per lo Studio della Sopravvivenza nell'infarto Miocardico. GISSI-3: effects of lisinopril and transdermal glyceryl trinitrate singly and together on 6-week mortality and ventricular function after acute myocardial infarction. Lancet. 1994;343:1115–22.

41. ISIS-4: a randomised factorial trial assessing early oral captopril, oral mononitrate, and intravenous magnesium sulphate in 58,050 patients with suspected acute myocardial infarction. ISIS-4 (Fourth International Study of Infarct Survival) Collaborative Group. Lancet. 1995;345:669.

42. The ESPRIM trial: short-term treatment of acute myocardial infarction with molsidomine. European Study of Prevention of Infarct with Molsidomine (ESPRIM) Group. Lancet. 1994;344:91–7.

43. Ren Z, Yang Q, Floten HS, Furnary AP, Yim AP, He GW. ATP-sensitive potassium channel openers may mimic the effects of hypoxic preconditioning on the coronary artery. Ann Thorac Surg. 2001;71:642–7.

44. Kitakaze M, Asakura M, Kim J, Shintani Y, Asanuma H, Hamasaki T, et al. for the J-WIND Investigators. Human atrial natriuretic peptide and nicorandil as adjuncts to reperfusion treatment for acute myocardial infarction (J-WIND): two randomised trials. Lancet. 2007;370:1483–93.

45. Iwakura K, Ito H, Okamura A, Yasushi Koyama Y, Date M, Higuchi Y, et al. Nicorandil treatment in patients with acute myocardial infarction. A meta-analysis. Circ J. 2009;73:925–31.
46. Zaza A, Belardinelli L, Shryock JC. Pathophysiology and pharmacology of the cardiac late sodium current. Pharmacol Ther. 2008;119:326–39.
47. Morrow D, Scirica B, Karwatowska E, Murphy E, Budja A, Varshavsky S, et al. Effects of ranolazine on recurrent cardiovascular events in patients with non–ST-elevation acute coronary syndromes he MERLIN-TIMI 36 randomized trial. JAMA. 2007;297:1775–83.
48. Wilson S, Scirica B, Braunwald E, Murphy S, Karwatowska E, Buros L, Chaitman B, Morrow D. Observations from the randomized, double-blind, placebo-controlled MERLIN–TIMI(metabolic efficiency with ranolazine for less ischemia in non–ST-segment elevation acute coronary syndromes) 36 trial. J Am Coll Cardiol. 2009;53:1510–6.
49. Kantor PF, Lucien A, Kozak R, Lopaschuk GD. The antianginal drug trimetazidine shifts cardiac energy metabolism from fatty acid oxidation to glucose oxidation by inhibiting mitochondrial long-chain 3-ketoacyl coenzyme a thiolase. Circ Res. 2000;86:580–8.
50. The EMIP-FR Group. European Myocardial Infarction Project--Free Radicals. Effect of 48-h intravenous trimetazidine on short- and long-term outcomes of patients with acute myocardial infarction, with and without thrombolytic therapy; A double-blind, placebo-controlled, randomized trial. Eur Heart J. 2000;18:1537–46.
51. Fox K, Borer JS, Camm AJ, Danchin N, Ferrari R, Lopez-Sendon J, Steg PG, Tardif JC, Tavazzi L, Tendera M. Resting heart rate in cardiovascular disease. J Am Coll Cardiol. 2007;50:823–30.
52. Granger CB, Goldberg RJ, Dabbous O, Pieper KS, Eagle KA, Cannon CP, Van de Werf F, Avezum Á, Goodman SG, Flather MD, Fox KAA, for the Global Registry of Acute Coronary Events Investigators. Predictors of hospital mortality in the Global Registry of Acute Coronary Events. Arch Intern Med. 2003;163:2345–53.
53. Yan AT, Yan RT, Tan M, et al. Risk scores for risk stratification in acute coronary syndromes: useful but simpler is not necessarily better. Eur Heart J. 2007;28:1072–8.
54. Herman M, Donovan J, Tran M, et al. Use of beta-blockers and effects on heart rate and blood pressure post-acute coronary syndromes: are we on target? Am Heart J. 2009;158:378–85.
55. Hjalmarson A, Gilpin EA, Kjekshus J, Chieman G, Nicod P, Henning H, et al. Influence of heart rate on mortality after acute myocardial infarction. Am J Cardiol. 1990;65:547–53.

Chapter 2
Antiplatelet Therapy. New Potent P2Y$_{12}$ Inhibitors

Pablo Avanzas, Cesar Morís, and Peter Clemmensen

Introduction

Acute coronary syndromes are conditions characterized by the sudden onset of coronary insufficiency as a result of the thrombotic occlusion of one or more coronary arteries. Depending on the extent of coronary occlusion, acute myocardial ischemic states range from unstable angina (UA) to non-ST-segment elevation myocardial infarction (NSTEMI) and ST-segment elevation myocardial infarction (STEMI). Platelets play a key pathophysiologic role in the atherothrombotic process that leads to an ischemic event; platelet-rich thrombi are formed at sites of vessel wall injury [1]. Therefore, antiplatelet agents are the current standard of care for ACS.

P. Avanzas, MD, PhD, FESC (✉)
Department of Cardiology, Hospital Universitario
Central de Asturias, Oviedo, Spain
e-mail: avanzas@secardiologia.es

C. Morís, MD, PhD
Department of Cardiology, Universidad de Oviedo, Oviedo, Spain

P. Clemmensen, MD, PhD, FESC
Department of Cardiology, The Heart Center,
Rigshospitalet, University Hospital of Copenhagen,
Copenhagen, Denmark

P. Avanzas, P. Clemmensen (eds.), *Pharmacological Treatment*   31
of Acute Coronary Syndromes, Current Cardiovascular Therapy,
DOI 10.1007/978-1-4471-5424-2_2,
© Springer-Verlag London 2014

There have been significant important advances in both antithrombotic and antiplatelet therapies with newer agents demonstrating improved cardiovascular outcomes and reductions in complications from bleeding. This chapter provides an overview on the current status of antiplatelet agents, specifically the new potent $P2Y_{12}$ inhibitors.

Classification of Antiplatelet Agents

Antiplatelet agents interfere with a variety of platelet functions, including aggregation, release of granule contents and platelet-mediated vascular constriction. They can be classified according to their mechanism of action (Fig. 2.1) [2]:

- Aspirin blocks cyclooxygenase (prostaglandin H synthase), the enzyme that mediates the first step in the biosynthesis of prostaglandins and thromboxane (including TxA_2) from arachidonic acid [3].
- The $P2Y_{12}$ receptor blockers (Table 2.1), clopidogrel, prasugrel, ticagrelor, cangrelor and elinogrel block the binding of adenosine diphosphate (ADP) to the platelet receptor $P2Y_{12}$, thereby inhibiting activation of the glycoprotein (GP) IIb/IIIa complex and platelet aggregation [4].
- Anti-GP IIb/IIIa antibodies and receptor antagonists inhibit the final common pathway of platelet aggregation (the cross-bridging of platelets by fibrinogen binding to the GP IIb/IIIa receptor) and may also prevent adhesion to the vessel wall [5].

Aspirin

Aspirin (acetylsalicylic acid) was the first antiplatelet drug to be employed clinically. It is still recommended for treatment of patients with ACS today, in combination to another antiplatelet agents [6]. Aspirin exerts its action through an irreversible blockade of COX-1, the enzyme that catalyzes the synthesis of thromboxane A2 (TXA_2) from arachidonic acid through selective acetylation of a serine residue at position

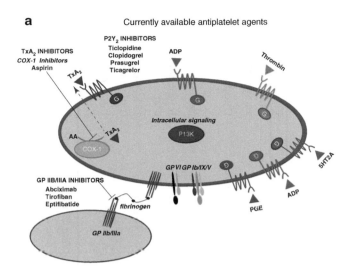

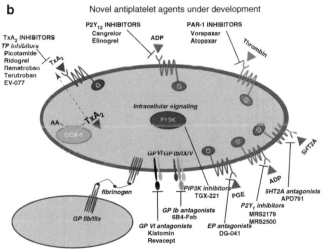

FIGURE 2.1 Sites of action of antiplatelet agents. (**a**) Currently available agents for acute coronary syndromes or percutaneous coronary intervention. (**b**) Novel antiplatelet agents under development. *AA* arachidonic acid, *ADP* adenosine diphosphate, *COX-1* cyclooxygenase-1, *EP* prostaglandin receptor, *G* g-protein, *GP* glycoprotein, *PG* prostanglandin, *PAR-1* platelet protease-activated receptor-1, *PI3K* phosphatidylinositol 3-kinase, *TP* thromboxane receptor, *TxA$_2$* thromboxane A$_2$ (Reprinted with permission from Ferreiro and Angiolillo [2])

TABLE 2.1 Pharmacological properties of P2Y$_{12}$ inhibitors

	Clopidogrel	Prasugrel	Ticagrelor	Cangrelor[a]	Elinogrel[a]
Drug class	Thienopyridine	Thienopyridine	Cyclopentyl triazopyrimidine	ATP analogue	Direct P2Y$_{12}$ antagonist
Metabolic conversion	Prodrug	Prodrug	Direct acting	Direct acting	Direct acting
Reversibility	No	No	Yes	Yes	Yes
Available formulation	Oral	Oral	Oral	Intravenous	Intravenous and oral
Half-life	7 h	3.5 h	12 h	10 min	12 h (Oral) 60 min (intravenous)
Duration of action	5–10 days	5–10 days	1 day	1 h	1 day (Oral) 2 h (intravenous)

[a]Cangrelor and elinogrel are investigational agents and not approved for clinical use at the time of preparation of this manuscript

529 (Ser529) [7, 8]. TXA$_2$ causes changes in platelet shape and enhances recruitment and aggregation of platelets through its binding to thromboxane and prostaglandin endoperoxide (TP) receptors. Therefore, aspirin decreases platelet activation and aggregation processes mediated by TP receptor pathways [9].

Aspirin is a cornerstone in the treatment of CVD [10]. The safety and efficacy of the drug has been evaluated in several populations, ranging from apparently healthy individuals at low risk of suffering cardiovascular events to high-risk patients presenting with ACS. Numerous clinical trials have demonstrated that aspirin is effective both in the acute treatment and in long-term secondary prevention of ACS [11, 12]. A strong evidence of aspirin benefit in cardiovascular diseases comes from a metaanalysis of 287 randomised trials of antiplatelet therapy for prevention of death, myocardial infarction, and stroke in high risk patients. The Antithrombotic Trialists' Collaboration [12] reviewed the effect of antiplatelet therapy, mostly aspirin (in doses ranging from 75 to 1,500 mg daily), in patients considered to be at high annual risk of vascular events because of evidence of pre-existing disease (previous occlusive event or predisposing condition). Overall, allocation to antiplatelet therapy reduced the combined outcome of any serious vascular event by about one quarter; nonfatal myocardial infarction was reduced by one third, nonfatal stroke by one quarter, and vascular mortality by one sixth (with no apparent adverse effect on other deaths).

In the ACS setting, an initial loading dose of 150–300 mg of uncoated aspirin should be given as soon as possible to any patient [13, 14]. At this dose, aspirin produces a rapid antithrombotic effect due to immediate and almost complete inhibition of thromboxane A$_2$ production. Aspirin should preferably be given orally (150–300 mg) -recommend chewing during the acute event-, to ensure complete inhibition of TXA$_2$-dependent platelet aggregation, but may be given intravenously in patients who are unable to swallow. There is little clinical data on the optimal i.v. dosage, but pharmacological data suggest that a lower dose range than that required for oral administration may avoid inhibition of prostacyclin. Therefore a bolus dose ranging from 80 to150 mg i.v. aspirin should be recommended.

P2Y$_{12}$ Receptor Antagonists

Adenosine diphosphate exerts its effects on platelets via the P2Y$_1$ and P2Y$_{12}$ receptors. Although both receptors are needed for aggregation, activation of the P2Y$_{12}$ pathway plays the principal role, leading to sustained platelet aggregation and stabilization of the platelet aggregate [2, 15]. P2Y$_{12}$ receptor inhibitors (Table 2.1) are recommended for prevention of ischemic events in both the acute and long-term phases of treatment, as will be described in details below. Clopidogrel has gained global recognition and is already widely used as described in more detail in Chap. 5. Two new agents (prasugrel and ticagrelor) are available as alternatives for use in place of clopidogrel, and two other agents (cangrelor and elinogrel) are also on the horizon.

Clopidogrel

Clopidogrel is a thienopyridine derivative that inhibits platelet aggregation. It is administered orally and maximal bioavailability occurs when it is taken after meals. Clopidogrel is a prodrug that requires metabolization in the liver through a double oxidation process mediated by several cytochrome P450 (CYP) isoforms, to be converted finally into its active metabolite, which irreversibly blocks the ADP P2Y$_{12}$ platelet receptor [16]. Due to the irreversible blockade of the P2Y$_{12}$ receptor [17, 18], clopidogrel effects last for the whole lifespan of the platelet (7–10 days).

Dual antiplatelet therapy with aspirin and clopidogrel is recommended per guidelines for patients with ACS, including those with UA or NSTEMI, STEMI and for patients undergoing PCI [13, 14]. This recommendation is based on the findings of several large-scale trials that have shown a clear benefit of adjunctive treatment with clopidogrel in addition to aspirin in preventing recurrent atherothrombotic events (Table 2.2) [6, 19–24]. Despite these evident clinical benefits, a substantial number of patients may continue to have recurrent cardiovascular events. Accumulating observations have shown certain clinically significant limitations associated to clopidogrel use, such us slower onset of action when compared with the more recently introduced antiplatelet drugs and variability in individual response [17, 18]. Inter-individual variation can result in coronary ischemia and stent thrombosis despite double antiplatelet therapy [25]. The reasons for variation in response are multifactorial and include genetic, cellular and clinical factors (Fig. 2.2). To overcome the drawbacks of clopidogrel, new potent potent P2Y$_{12}$ receptor inhibitors have been developed in the recent years.

Prasugrel

Prasugrel is an oral, irreversible thienopyridine inhibitor of the platelet P2Y$_{12}$ ADP receptor and, like clopidogrel, a prodrug that is rapidly absorbed and requires in vivo metabolism to form its active metabolite (Fig. 2.3) [26]. Prasugrel has a faster onset of action than clopidogrel, and leads to greater platelet inhibition with less variability of response. This superiority is mainly due to its greater bioavailability, which is related to its simpler metabolism that allows the more rapid and extensive formation of its ex vivo clopidogrel-equipotent active metabolite. Furthermore, the genetic polymorphisms that limit the effectiveness of clopidogrel do not seem to affect prasugrel. Prasugrel treated patients requiring surgery warrant a 7 day washout period to minimize bleeding complications.

The Trial to Assess Improvement in Therapeutic Outcomes by Optimizing Platelet Inhibition with Prasugrel–Thrombolysis in Myocardial Infarction (TRITON-TIMI 38)

TABLE 2.2 Efficacy results from major clopidogrel studies

Study[a] (setting)	Treatments	Primary efficacy endpoints	Follow-up	Primary end point data [% (p-value)]
CAPRIE [19] (atherosclerotic disease)	CLO 75 mg/day (n = 9,599) vs ASA 325 mg/day (n=9,586)	Composite outcome cluster of ischaemic stroke, MI or vascular death	1.9 years	5.32 vs 5.83 (0.043)
CURE [20] (ACS without ST elevation)	CLO 300 mg LD, then 75 mg/day (n=6,259) plus ASA 75–325 mg/day vs ASA alone (n=6,303)	Composite of death from CV causes, non-fatal MI or stroke	3–12 months	9.3 vs 11.4 (<0.001)
CLARITY [21] (fibrinolysis after STEMI)	CLO 300 mg LD, then 75 mg/day plus ASA 150–325 mg LD then 75–162 mg/day (n=1,752) vs ASA alone (n=1,739)	Composite of occluded infarct-related artery (defined by a TIMI flow grade of 0 or 1) on angiography, death or recurrent MI before angiography	30 days	15.0 vs 21.7 (<0.001)
COMMIT [22] (acute MI)	CLO 75 mg/day (n = 22,961) plus ASA 162 mg/day vs ASA alone (n=22,891)	Composite of death, re-infarction or stroke; and death from any cause during the scheduled treatment period	4 weeks	Composite: 9.2 vs 10.1 (0.002) Death: 7.5 vs 8.1 (0.03)

| CREDOS [23] (ACS with PCI) | CLO 300 mg LD (n=1,053) or PL (n=1,063) 3–24 h before PCI. Thereafter, all pts received CLO 75 mg/day through d 28. From days 29 through 12 months, pts in the LD group received CLO 75 mg/day, and those in the control group received PL. Both groups received ASA throughout the study | 1 year end point: composite of death, MI and stroke in the ITT population 28 days endpoint; composite of death, MI or urgent TVR in the per-protocol population | 1 year 28 days | 8.5 vs 11.5 (0.02) 6.8 vs 8.3 (0.23) |
| CHARISMA [24] (CVD or multiple risk factors) | CLO 75 months/day plus low-dose ASA 75–162 mg/day or PL plus low-dose ASA | Composite MI, stroke or death from CV causes | 28 months | 6.8 vs 7.3 (0.22) |

Reprinted with permission from: Angiolillo [6]

ACS acute coronary syndrome, *ASA* aspirin (acetylsalicylic acid), *CLO* clopidogrel, *CV* cardiovascular, *CVD* cardiovascular disease, *ITT* intent to treat, *LD* loading dose, *MI* myocardial infarction, *PCI* percutaneous coronary intervention, *PL* placebo, *pts* patients, *STEMI*-ST segment elevation myocardial infarction, *TIMI* Thrombolysis In Myocardial Infarction, *TVR* target vessel revascularization

[a] Refer to Table 2.1 for full names of each trial

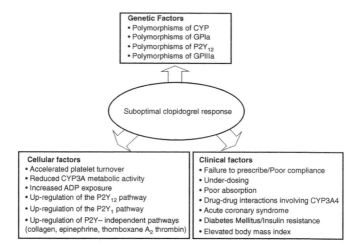

FIGURE 2.2 Proposed mechanisms leading to variability in individual responsiveness to clopidogrel (Reprinted with permission from Angiolillo et al. [17])

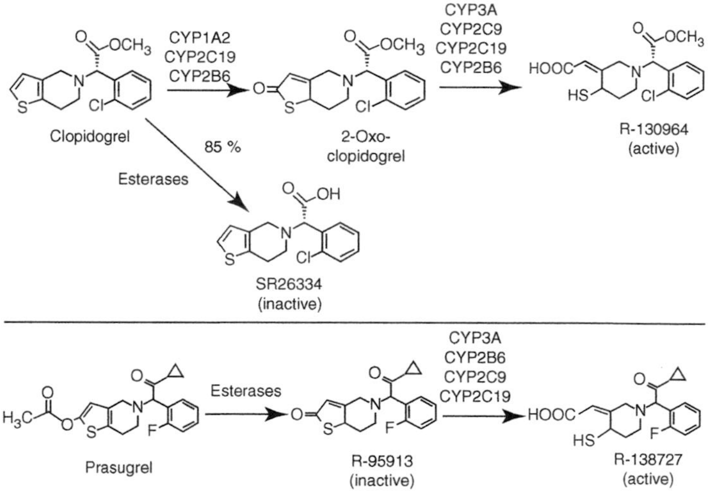

FIGURE 2.3 Structures and primary metabolic pathways for prasugrel and clopidogrel

[27] compared the use of prasugrel (60-mg loading dose and maintenance dose of 10 mg/day) with clopidogrel (300-mg loading dose followed by a daily 75-mg maintenance dose) in 13,608 patients with moderate to high risk of ACS for whom PCI was scheduled (26 % STEMI; 74 % unstable angina or NSTEMI). All patients received aspirin at a dose of 81 mg daily. For patients with unstable angina or NSTEMI, the coronary anatomy had to be known before randomization. Thus, in the majority of cases both clopidogrel and prasugrel were given after coronary angiography. Patients were followed-up over a period of 6–5 months. The primary efficacy endpoint (CV death, non-fatal MI or non-fatal stroke) occurred in 12.1 and 9.9 % of the clopidogrel and prasugrel groups respectively (HR 0.81 [95 % CI: 0.73–0.90,]; P < 0.001). Prasugrel reduced MI rates (9.7 and 7.4 % respectively; P < 0.001) and urgent target-vessel revascularization (3.7 and 2.5 % respectively; P < 0.001). Prasugrel also decreased the likelihood of stent thrombosis (2.4 and 1.1 %; P < 0.001), in patients treated with BMS only (HR 0.52 [0.35–0.77]; P < 0.001) and in those who received at least one DES (HR 0.43 [0.28–0.66]; P < 0.001). Congruent with the higher antiplatelet activity, the prasugrel group also had higher major bleeding rates (2.4 % vs 1.8 %; hazard ratio [HR], 1.32; 95 % CI, 1.03–1.68; P = 0.03). Life-threatening bleeding (1.4 and 0.9 % respectively; p = 0.01), nonfatal bleeding (1.1 and 0.9 % respectively; p = 0.23) and fatal bleeding (0.4 and 0.1 % respectively; p = 0.002) were more common with prasugrel than clopidogrel. Three high-risk subgroups with lesser net clinical efficacy and higher rates of bleeding were found in a post hoc analysis: patients ≥75 year old, patients weighing ≤60 kg and patients with a history of stroke or transient ischemic attack. After excluding high-risk patients, no significant difference emerged in the rate of major bleeding between prasugrel and clopidogrel (HR 1.24 [0.91–1.69]; P = 0.17).

Additional subanalyses of the TRITON TIMI 38 suggest that the magnitude of the effect was enhanced in patients presenting with STEMI treated with primary or delayed PCI [28] and diabetic patients [29]. Among patients (n = 3,534) undergoing PCI for STEMI [28], 6.5 and 9.5 % of the prasu-grel and clopidogrel arms respectively met the primary end-point after 30 days (HR 0.68 [0.54–0.87]; p = 0.0017). Prasugrel's superiority persisted for 15 months (10.0 and 12.4 %; HR 0.79 [0.65–0.97]; p = 0.0221). On multivariable adjustment for baseline differences, prasugrel reduced 30-day rates of the primary endpoint (HR 0.81 [0.66–0.99]; p = 0.0488), a secondary composite endpoint of CV death, MI or urgent target vessel revascularisation (6.7 and 8.8 % respectively; HR 0.75 [0.59–0.96]; p = 0.0205) and stent thrombosis (1.2 and 2.4 % respectively; HR 0.49 [0.28–0.84]; p = 0.0084) compared with clopidogrel. Patients with diabetes mellitus (DM) had greater benefit compared with nondiabetic patients when dual antiplatelet therapy with prasugrel was used. In a sub-analysis of the TRITON-TIMI 38 study [29], prasugrel use was more efficacious compared with clopidogrel in reducing the ischemic event rates in both diabetics and nondiabetics, with greater reduction in diabetics. The rate of primary end-point among patients without DM was 9.2 % versus 10.6 % (HR, 0.86; P = 0.02) and was 12.2 % versus 17.0 % among patients with DM (HR, 0.70; P < 0.001). The TIMI major hem-orrhage rates were similar among patients with DM for clopi-dogrel and prasugrel (2.6 % vs 2.5 %; HR, 1.06; P = 0.81). This suggests that the greater antiplatelet activity produced by prasugrel resulted in higher net clinical benefit in patients with DM when compared with patients without DM.

The TRILOGY-ACS study examined the use of prasugrel versus clopidogrel in 9,326 patients with unstable angina or NSTEMI who were selected for a final treatment strategy of medical management [30] Additionally, patients were required to have at least one of the following risk factors: an age of ≥60 years, the presence of diabetes mellitus, previous MI or previous revascularization with either PCI or CABG. Randomization was carried out at a median of more than 4 days after admission. Prasugrel was given with a loading dose of 30 mg and a maintenance dose of 10 mg/day in patients less than 75 years or 5 mg/day for those ≥75 years or weighed <60 kg; clopidogrel was given with a 300 mg loading dose and

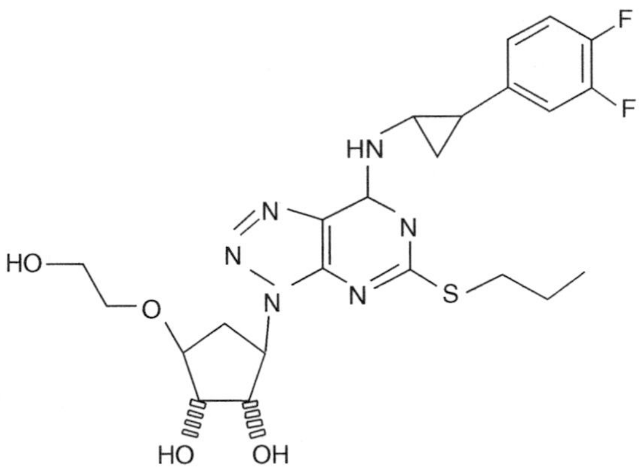

FIGURE 2.4 Chemical structure of ticagrelor

a 75 mg/day maintenance dose. The primary efficacy end point was a composite of death from cardiovascular causes, nonfatal MI, or nonfatal stroke among patients under the age of 75 years. Among the primary cohort of patients aged <75 years and at a median follow-up of 17.1 months, there was no significant between-group difference in the rate of the primary endpoint (death from vascular causes, MI or stroke), which occurred in 13.9 % of patients receiving prasugrel compared with 16.0 % of patients receiving clopidogrel (HR 0.91 [95 % CI 0.79, 1.05]; P=0.21). Similar results were observed in the overall population (18.7 % vs 20.3 %; HR 0.96 [95 % CI 0.86, 1.07]; P=0.45), albeit with a significant decrease in the total number of events (first, and recurrent) favoring prasugrel.

Ticagrelor

Ticagrelor (Fig. 2.4) is a novel oral direct-acting platelet blocker that binds reversibly to the P2Y$_{12}$ receptor [31]. Due to the short half-life, it is dosed twice daily for maintenance therapy. Platelet function typically normalizes within 24–48 h after termination of therapy [32]. Ticagrelor-treated patients requiring surgery warrant a minimum of a 5 day washout period to minimize bleeding complications. It is contraindicated in patients at high risk of bleeding, with prior hemorrhagic stroke and severe hepatic dysfunction. Because ticagrelor is metabolized by CYP3A4/5 enzymes, the prescribing information for ticagrelor recommends that patients taking ticagrelor should avoid the use of strong inhibitors or inducers of CYP3A [2].

PLATO is multicenter, double-blind, randomized trial, that compared ticagrelor (180-mg loading dose, 90 mg twice daily thereafter) and clopidogrel (300-to-600-mg loading dose, 75 mg daily thereafter) for the prevention of cardiovascular events in 18,624 patients admitted to the hospital with an acute coronary syndrome, with or without ST-segment elevation [33]. In contrast to TRITON-TIMI 38, in PLATO patients pretreated with clopidogrel were eligible for enrollment, and randomization generally occurred before defining coronary anatomy to reflect current practice patterns.

At 12 months, the primary end point – a composite of death from vascular causes, myocardial infarction, or stroke – had occurred in 9.8 % of patients receiving ticagrelor as compared with 11.7 % of those receiving clopidogrel (hazard ratio, 0.84; 95 % confidence interval [CI], 0.77–0.92; P < 0.001,). Predefined hierarchical testing of secondary end points showed significant differences in the rates of other composite end points, as well as myocardial infarction alone (5.8 % in the ticagrelor group vs. 6.9 % in the clopidogrel group, P = 0.005) and death from vascular causes (4.0 % vs. 5.1 %, P = 0.001) but not stroke alone (1.5 % vs. 1.3 %, P = 0.22). The rate of death from any cause was also reduced with ticagrelor (4.5 %, vs. 5.9 % with clopidogrel; P < 0.001). No significant difference in the rates of major bleeding was found between the ticagrelor and clopidogrel groups (11.6 and 11.2 %, respectively; P = 0.43), but ticagrelor was associated with a higher rate of major bleeding not related to coronary-artery bypass grafting (4.5 % vs. 3.8 %, P = 0.03), including more instances of fatal intracranial bleeding and fewer of fatal bleeding of other types.

Of remark, the benefit of ticagrelor was consistent across different subgroup analyses, such as patients with an initial conservative approach with noninvasive treatment strategy [34], patients undergoing a planned invasive strategy [35], those undergoing CABG [36] and in patients with chronic kidney disease [37].

In contrast to results in TRITON, where three high-risk subgroups with lesser net clinical efficacy and higher rates of bleeding were identified in a post hoc analysis, in PLATO there weren't any specific subgroups that emerged to have higher bleeding potential with ticagrelor, including patients with prior transient ischemic/ischemic stroke. However, several non hematological safety end points, which have been associated with higher discontinuation rates, have been observed with ticagrelor. These include increased levels of creatinine and uric acid during treatment and higher rates of dyspnea and ventricular pauses, compared with clopidogrel.

In the PLATO trial, a prespecified subgroup analysis showed a significant interaction between treatment and region ($P = 0.045$), with less effect of ticagrelor in North America than in the rest of the world. Results of 2 independently performed analyses identified an underlying statistical interaction with aspirin maintenance dose as a possible explanation for the regional difference. The lowest risk of cardiovascular death, myocardial infarction, or stroke with ticagrelor compared with clopidogrel is associated with a low maintenance dose of concomitant aspirin. Current prescribing information for ticagrelor includes a warning to avoid aspirin doses >100 mg in patients receiving the drug [38].

Notably, PLATO was the first study to demonstrate a reduction of overall mortality with a new P2Y$_{12}$ receptor inhibitor in comparison to clopidogrel although the study was not powered to detect differences in the mortality rate. Several explanations for the mortality benefits with ticagrelor beyond its superior antiplatelet effects have been postulated including its potential to modulate endogenous adenosine concentration with subsequent favourable vascular effects [39].

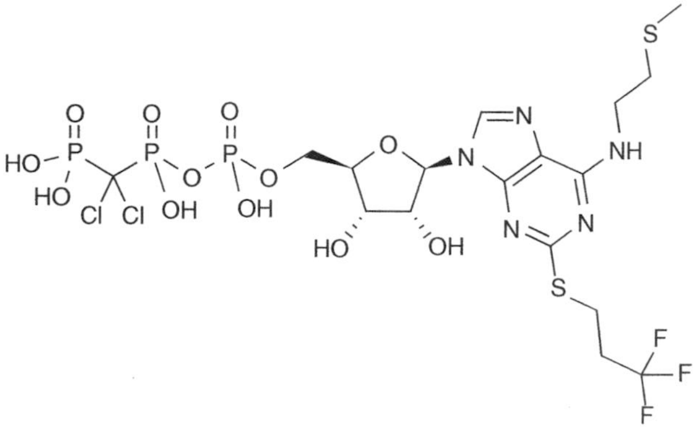

FIGURE2.5 Chemical structure of cangrelor

Cangrelor

Cangrelor (previously known as AR-C69931MX, Fig. 2.5) is an adenosine triphosphate analog that has a potent, direct, and reversible $P2Y_{12}$ receptor inhibition. It is the first $P2Y_{12}$ inhibitor that is available in intravenous form. It acts directly on the $P2Y_{12}$ receptor without the need for hepatic conversion to an active metabolite, in contrast to prasugrel and clopidogrel [40]. It has a rapid onset of action (few seconds) after the administration of a bolus dose. It also has a short half-life of 3–6 min and its platelet inhibitory effect is reversed within 30–60 min after discontinuation of the drug infusion [41]. After binding to the $P2Y_{12}$ receptor, Cangrelor is rapidly inactivated by an ADPase located on the surface of vascular endothelial cells [42].

Cangrelor has been compared to either clopidogrel or placebo in three randomized trials that included patients with non-ST elevation coronary syndrome (NSTEACS) and evaluated 48-h outcomes [2]. The CHAMPION (Cangrelor versus standard tHerapy to Achieve optimal Management of Platelet InhibitiON) program initially included the CHAMPION-PCI [43] and the CHAMPION-PLATFORM [44] trials, which evaluated mostly ACS patients undergoing

PCI, and were terminated before completion because of an interim analysis showing insufficient evidence of clinical effectiveness of cangrelor (bolus 30 µg/kg plus infusion of 4 µg/kg/min for the duration of the PCI procedure, with a minimum infusion duration of 2 h and a maximum of 4 h). Differences in trial designs and definition of study end points may have contributed to failure to show superiority in terms of reduction of adverse ischemic outcomes of cangrelor over clopidogrel in CHAMPION-PCI (n = 8,716), and over placebo in CHAMPION-PLATFORM (n = 5,362) trials. The CHAMPION-PHOENIX trial [45] randomly assigned 11,145 patients who were undergoing either urgent or elective PCI and were receiving guideline-recommended therapy to receive a bolus and infusion of cangrelor or to receive a loading dose of 600 mg or 300 mg of clopidogrel. The primary efficacy end point was a composite of death, myocardial infarction, ischemia-driven revascularization, or stent thrombosis at 48 h after randomization. The primary safety end point was severe bleeding at 48 h. The rate of the primary efficacy end point was 4.7 % in the cangrelor group and 5.9 % in the clopidogrel group (adjusted odds ratio with cangrelor, 0.78; 95 % confidence interval [CI], 0.66–0.93; P = 0.005). The rate of the primary safety end point was 0.16 % in the cangrelor group and 0.11 % in the clopidogrel group (odds ratio, 1.50; 95 % CI, 0.53–4.22; P = 0.44). Stent thrombosis developed in 0.8 % of the patients in the cangrelor group and in 1.4 % in the clopidogrel group (odds ratio, 0.62; 95 % CI, 0.43–0.90; P = 0.01). The rates of adverse events related to the study treatment were low in both groups, though transient dyspnea occurred significantly more frequently with cangrelor than with clopidogrel (1.2 % vs. 0.3 %). The benefit from cangrelor with respect to the primary end point was consistent across multiple prespecified subgroups. Taking in account efficacy results in the CHAMPION program and the fact cangrelor has not been directly compared to either ticagrelor or prasugrel, we believe that the potential role of cangrelor in reducing isquemic events in ACS patients remains to be determined.

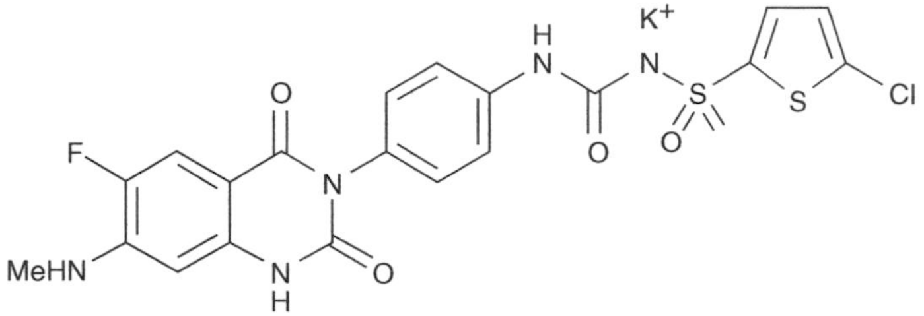

FIGURE 2.6 Chemical structure of elinogrel

However, cangrelor may still have a role, due to its pharma-cological properties, as a bridging strategy in the setting of patients requiring surgery but who require treatment with a P2Y$_{12}$ inhibitor to prevent thrombotic complications.

The BRIDGE (Maintenance of platelet inhiBition with cangreloR after dIscontinuation of thienopyriDines in patients undergoing surGEry) trial was a prospective, ran-domized double-blind, placebo controlled, multicenter trial in patients (n=210) with an ACS or treated with a coronary stent on a thienopyridine awaiting CABG to receive either placebo or cangrelor at a dose (0.75 µg/kg/min) identified in dose-finding phase of the trial [2, 46]. Among patients who discontinue thienopyridine therapy prior to cardiac surgery, the use of cangrelor compared with placebo resulted in a higher rate of maintenance of platelet inhibition. Therefore, cangrelor may represent a future option for bridging therapy in patients with ACS or treated with coronary stents who require surgery.

Elinogrel

Elinogrel, a quinazoline-2,4-dione (Fig. 2.6), is a potent, revers-ible, ADP receptor antagonist that is available in an oral and intravenous formulation [47]. Maximum platelet inhibition is achieved within 15 min of intravenous administration result-ing in more rapid platelet inhibition effects than any other oral antiplatelet drugs. Elinogrel has a plasma half-life of approximately 12 h. Its direct mode of action does not require metabolic activation or conversion into an active drug leading to reduced variability in drug response compared to clopidogrel. Polymorphisms of genes codifying hepatic cytochrome P450 isoenzymes do not seem to play a role in the elinogrel response rate [48]. The compound is cleared to a similar extent through the kidney and the liver [49].

Elinogrel has been tested in two phase 2 studies in patients with ST- elevation myocardial infarction (STEMI) and in patients with stable CAD undergoing PCI.

The ERASE-MI trial [50] examined the safety and tolerability elinogrel versus placebo when administered to STEMI patients before primary PCI. Patients were randomized to escalating doses (10, 20, 40, and 60 mg) of elinogrel administered as a single intravenous bolus before the start of the diagnostic angiogram preceding primary PCI or placebo. All patients received a 600-mg clopidogrel loading dose, followed by a second 300-mg clopidogrel loading dose 4 h after PCI. The major outcome, in-hospital bleeding, was assessed with the Thrombolysis in Myocardial Infarction and Global Strategics to Open Occluded Coronary Arteries bleeding scales. Seventy patients were randomized in the dose-escalation study, but the dose-confirmation phase was not started because the trial was prematurely terminated for administrative reasons. The incidence of bleeding events was infrequent and appeared to be similar in patients treated with all doses of elinogrel versus placebo.

The INNOVATE-PCI trial [51] evaluated the safety, efficacy, and tolerability of elinogrel in patients undergoing non-urgent percutaneous coronary intervention. Patients (n = 652) received either 300 or 600 mg of clopidogrel pre-percutaneous coronary intervention followed by 75 mg daily or 80 or 120 mg of IV elinogrel followed by 50, 100, or 150 mg oral elinogrel twice daily. In comparison with clopidogrel, intravenous and oral elinogrel therapy did not significantly increase thrombolysis in myocardial infarction major or minor bleeding, although bleeding requiring medical attention was more common. The significance of these findings will need to be more definitively determined in future phase 3 studies.

Glycoprotein IIB/IIIA Inhibitors

Platelet GPIIb/IIIa complex is intimately involved in platelet aggregation. GPIIb/IIIa changes its conformation following platelet activation, becomes a receptor for fibrinogen, and the fibrinogen links adjacent platelets together. The GPIIb/IIIa antagonists block the interaction of fibrinogen with the activated GPIIb/IIIa complex. These drugs do not prevent the initial activation of platelets by the various agents that bring this about, but block the final common pathway in the aggregation process [52]. There are available three different GPIs currently approved for clinical use: abciximab, eptifibatide, and tirofiban These drugs are only available for intravenous use and have a rapid onset of action and a very potent inhibitory effect on platelets, so their use is restricted to the acute phase of treatment [5]. Importantly, the efficacy of these agents correlates directly with the severity and the risk of ACS, reaching their maximal benefit in high risk ACS patients undergoing PCI [53].

In NSTEMI patients, GP IIb/IIIa inhibitors may be considered in the catheterization laboratory in high-risk patients, in patients with significant intracoronary thrombus burden, or in the absence of timely antiplatelet pre-treatment. In these cases, the strongest evidence supports the use of abciximab. Also, in the setting of STEMI, GP IIb/IIIa inhibitors should be considered for bailout therapy if there is angiographic evidence of massive thrombus, slow or no-reflow or a thrombotic complication. Routine upstream therapy with GP IIb/IIIa inhibitors is not recommended at present [13, 14].

Finally, we have to keep in mind that many trials evaluating GP IIb/IIIa inhibitors' efficacy were performed before in the era in which the new $P2Y_{12}$ inhibiting agents prasugrel and ticagrelor were not available and the regimens of clopidogrel that are currently being used (e.g., pretreatment, high loading doses) were not part of the standard of care. Therefore, the role of GP IIb/IIIa inhibitors in today's clinical practice is diminished significantly.

Future Perspectives and Conclusions

Despite the known benefit of dual antiplatelet therapy in patients with ACS, a substantial percentage of patients still present recurrent atherothrombotic events, leading to the development of newer and more potent antiplatelet agents, some of which have already been approved for clinical use, such as prasugrel and ticagrelor [54]. The potent antiplatelet agents prasugrel and ticagrelor are now the treatment of choice for ACS patients. In the current ESC ACS guidelines, clopidogrel is only recommended for patients who cannot receive ticagrelor or prasugrel. The choice of ticagrelor or prasugrel for a given ACS patients may be difficult, and stresses the need for clear institutional or regional protocol, but both are recommended with equal weight in the guidelines [13, 14], particularly in the STEMI setting. It emerges that prasugrel is mostly used in STEMI or in NSTEMI with very rapid access to invasive evaluation, as a consequence of the recommendation to have the coronary anatomy well defined prior to first dose. . By virtue of the PLATO study design, ticagrelor does not have this same limitation in use. Large scale studies with head-to head comparisons between prasugrel and ticagrelor are unlikely to be performed, so each institution must have a well defined strategy of individualized treatment or a common drug for all patients without contraindications.

References

1. Furie B, Furie BC. Mechanisms of thrombus formation. N Engl J Med. 2008;359:938–49.
2. Ferreiro JL, Angiolillo DJ. New directions in antiplatelet therapy. Circ Cardiovasc Interv. 2012;5(3):433–45.
3. Patrono C. Aspirin as an antiplatelet drug. N Engl J Med. 1994; 330:1287.
4. Foster CJ, Prosser DM, Agans JM, et al. Molecular identification and characterization of the platelet ADP receptor targeted by thienopyridine antithrombotic drugs. J Clin Invest. 2001;107:1591.

5. Kristensen SD, Würtz M, Grove EL, De Caterina R, Huber K, Moliterno DJ, Neumann FJ. Contemporary use of glycoprotein IIb/IIIa inhibitors. Thromb Haemost. 2012;107(2):215–24.
6. Angiolillo DJ. The evolution of antiplatelet therapy in the treatment of acute coronary syndromes: from aspirin to the present day. Drugs. 2012;72(16):2087–116.
7. May JA, Heptinstall S, Cole AT, Hawkey CJ. Platelet responses to several agonists and combinations of agonists in whole blood: a placebo controlled comparison of the effects of a once daily dose of plain aspirin 300 mg, plain aspirin 75 mg and enteric coated aspirin 300 mg, in man. Thromb Res. 1997;88:183–92.
8. Perneby C, Wallén NH, Rooney C, Fitzgerald D, Hjemdahl P. Dose- and time-dependent antiplatelet effects of aspirin. Thromb Haemost. 2006;95:652–8.
9. Patrono C, García Rodríguez LA, Landolfi R, Baigent C. Low-dose aspirin for the prevention of atherothrombosis. N Engl J Med. 2005; 353:2373–83.
10. Fuster V, Badimon L, Badimon JJ, et al. The pathogenesis of coronary artery disease and the acute coronary syndromes (part 1). N Engl J Med. 1992;326:242–50.
11. ISIS-2 (Second International Study of Infarct Survival) Collaborative Group. Randomized trial of intravenous streptokinase, oral aspirin, both, or neither among 17,187 cases of suspected acute myocardial infarction: ISIS-2. ISIS-2 (Second International Study of Infarct Survival) Collaborative Group. J Am Coll Cardiol. 1988;12:3A–13.
12. Antithrombotic Trialists' Collaboration. Collaborative meta-analysis of randomised trials of antiplatelet therapy for prevention of death, myocardial infarction, and stroke in high risk patients. BMJ. 2002;324:71–86.
13. Task Force on the management of ST-segment elevation acute myocardial infarction of the European Society of Cardiology (ESC), Steg PG, James SK, Atar D, Badano LP, Blömstrom-Lundqvist C, Borger MA, Di Mario C, Dickstein K, Ducrocq G, Fernandez-Aviles F, Gershlick AH, Giannuzzi P, Halvorsen S, Huber K, Juni P, Kastrati A, Knuuti J, Lenzen MJ, Mahaffey KW, Valgimigli M, van't Hof A, Widimsky P, Zahger D. ESC Guidelines for the management of acute myocardial infarction in patients presenting with ST-segment elevation. Eur Heart J. 2012;33(20):2569–619.
14. Hamm CW, Bassand JP, Agewall S, Bax J, Boersma E, Bueno H, Caso P, Dudek D, Gielen S, Huber K, Ohman M, Petrie MC, Sonntag F, Uva MS, Storey RF, Wijns W, Zahger D, ESC Committee for Practice Guidelines. ESC Guidelines for the management of acute coronary syndromes in patients presenting without persistent ST-segment elevation: The Task Force for the management of acute coronary syndromes (ACS) in patients presenting without persistent

ST-segment elevation of the European Society of Cardiology (ESC). Eur Heart J. 2011;32(23):2999–3054.

15. Storey RF, Newby LJ, Heptinstall S. Effects of P2Y(1) and P2Y(12) receptor antagonists on platelet aggregation induced by different agonists in human whole blood. Platelets. 2001;12:443–7.

16. Verstraete M, Zoldhelyi P. Novel antithrombotic drugs in development. Drugs. 1995;49:856–84.

17. Angiolillo DJ, Fernandez-Ortiz A, Bernardo E, Alfonso F, Macaya C, Bass TA, et al. Variability in individual responsiveness to clopidogrel: clinical implications, management, and future perspectives. J Am Coll Cardiol. 2007;49:1505–16.

18. Ferreiro JL, Angiolillo DJ. Clopidogrel response variability: current status and future directions. Thromb Haemost. 2009;102:7–14.

19. CAPRIE SteeringCommittee. A randomised, blinded, trial of clopidogrel versus aspirin in patients at risk of ischacmic events (CAPRIE). Lancet. 1996;348:1329–39.

20. Yusuf S, Zhao F, Mehta SR, et al. Effects of clopidogrel in addition to aspirin in patients with acute coronary syndromes without ST-segment elevation. N Engl J Med. 2001;345:494–502.

21. Sabatine MS, Cannon CP, CLARITY-TIMI 28 Investigators, et al. Addition of clopidogrel to aspirin and fibrinolytic therapy for myo cardial infarction with ST-segment elevation. N Engl J Med. 2005; 352:1179–89.

22. Chen ZM, Jiang LX, Chen YP, et al. Addition of clopidogrel to aspirin in 45 852 patients with acute myocardial infarction: randomised placebo-controlled trial. Lancet. 2005;366:1607–21.

23. Steinhubl SR, Berger PB, CREDO Investigators, et al. Clopidogrel for the Reduction of Events During Observation. Early and sustained dual oral antiplatelet therapy following percutaneous coronary intervention: a randomized controlled trial. JAMA. 2002;288: 2411–20.

24. Bhatt DL, Fox KA, Hacke W, et al. CHARISMA Investigators: clopidogrel and aspirin versus aspirin alone for the prevention of atherothrombotic events. N Engl J Med. 2006;354:1706–17.

25. Wiviott SD, Antman EM, Braunwald E. Prasugrel. Circulation. 2010; 122:394–403.

26. Mega JL, Close SL, Wiviott SD, Shen L, Hockett RD, Brandt JT, Walker JR, Antman EM, Macias WL, Braunwald E, Sabatine MS. Cytochrome P450 genetic polymorphisms and the response to prasugrel: relationship to pharmacokinetic, pharmacodynamic, and clinical outcomes. Circulation. 2009;119(19):2553–60.

27. Wiviott SD, Braunwald E, McCabe CH, et al. Prasugrel versus clopidogrel in patients with acute coronary syndromes. N Engl J Med. 2007;357:2001–15.

28. Montalescot G, Wiviott SD, Braunwald E, et al. Prasugrel compared with clopidogrel in patients undergoing percutaneous coronary inter-

vention for STelevation myocardial infarction (TRITON-TIMI 38): double-blind, randomised controlled trial. Lancet. 2009;373:723–31.

29. Wiviott SD, Braunwald E, Angiolillo DJ, et al. Greater clinical benefit of more intensive oral antiplatelet therapy with prasugrel in patients with diabetes mellitus in the trial to assess improvement in therapeutic outcomes by optimizing platelet inhibition with prasugrel–Thrombolysis in Myocardial Infarction 38. Circulation. 2008;118(16):1626–36.

30. Roe MT, Armstrong PW, Fox KA, White HD, Prabhakaran D, Goodman SG, Cornel JH, Bhatt DL, Clemmensen P, Martinez F, Ardissino D, Nicolau JC, Boden WE, Gurbel PA, Ruzyllo W, Dalby AJ, McGuire DK, Leiva-Pons JL, Parkhomenko A, Gottlieb S, Topacio GO, Hamm C, Pavlides G, Goudev AR, Oto A, Tseng CD, Merkely B, Gasparovic V, Corbalan R, Cinteză M, McLendon RC, Winters KJ, Brown EB, Lokhnygina Y, Aylward PE, Huber K, Hochman JS, Ohman EM, TRILOGY ACS Investigators. Prasugrel versus clopidogrel for acute coronary syndromes without revascularization. N Engl J Med. 2012;367(14):1297–309.

31. Htun WW, Steinhubl SR. Ticagrelor: the first novel reversible $P2Y_{12}$ inhibitor. Expert Opin Pharmacother. 2013;14(2):237–45.

32. Gurbel PA, Bliden KP, Butler K, et al. Randomized double-blind assessment of the ONSET and OFFSET of the antiplatelet effects of ticagrelor versus clopidogrel in patients with stable coronary artery disease: the ONSET/OFFSET study. Circulation. 2009;120: 2577–85.

33. Wallentin L, Becker RC, Budaj A, Cannon CP, Emanuelsson H, Held C, Horrow J, Husted S, James S, Katus H, Mahaffey KW, Scirica BM, Skene A, Steg PG, Storey RF, Harrington RA, PLATO Investigators, Freij A, Thorsén M. Ticagrelor versus clopidogrel in patients with acute coronary syndromes. N Engl J Med. 2009;361(11): 1045–57.

34. James SK, Roe MT, Cannon CP, Cornel JH, Horrow J, Husted S, Katus H, Morais J, Steg PG, Storey RF, Stevens S, Wallentin L, Harrington RA, PLATO Study Group. Ticagrelor versus clopidogrel in patients with acute coronary syndromes intended for non-invasive management: substudy from prospective randomised PLATelet inhibition and patient Outcomes (PLATO) trial. BMJ. 2011;342:d3527.

35. Cannon CP, Harrington RA, James S, Ardissino D, Becker RC, Emanu-elsson H, Husted S, Katus H, Keltai M, Khurmi NS, Kontny F, Lewis BS, Steg PG, Storey RF, Wojdyla D, Wallentin L, PLATelet Inhibition and Patient Outcomes Investigators. Comparison of ticagrelor with clopidogrel in patients with a planned invasive strategy for acute coronary syndromes (PLATO): a randomised double-blind study. Lancet. 2010;375:283–93.

36. Held C, Asenblad N, Bassand JP, Becker RC, Cannon CP, Claeys MJ, Harrington RA, Horrow J, Husted S, James SK, Mahaffey KW, Nicolau JC, Scirica BM, Storey RF, Vintila M, Ycas J, Wallentin L. Ticagrelor versus clopidogrel in patients with acute coronary syndromes undergoing coronary artery bypass surgery: results from the PLATO (Platelet Inhi- bition and Patient Outcomes) trial. J Am Coll Cardiol. 2011;57:672–84.

37. James S, Budaj A, Aylward P, et al. Ticagrelor versus clopidogrel in acute coronary syndromes in relation to renal function: results from the Platelet Inhibition and Patient Outcomes (PLATO) trial. Circulation. 2010;122:1056–67.

38. Mahaffey KW, Wojdyla DM, Carroll K, Becker RC, Storey RF, Angiolillo DJ, Held C, Cannon CP, James S, Pieper KS, Horrow J, Harrington RA, Wallentin L, PLATO Investigators. Ticagrelor compared with clopidogrel by geographic region in the Platelet Inhibition and Patient Outcomes (PLATO) trial. Circulation. 2011;124: 544–54.

39. Wallentin L, Becker RC, James SK, Harrington RA. The PLATO trial reveals further opportunities to improve outcomes in patients with acute coronary syndrome. Thromb Haemost. 2011;105: 760–2.

40. Tan GM, Lam YY, Yan BP. Novel platelet ADP P2Y$_{12}$ inhibitors in the treatment of acute coronary syndrome. Cardiovasc Ther. 2012; 30(4):e167–73.

41. Wang K, Zhou X, Zhou Z, et al. Sustained coronary artery recanalization with adjunctive infusion of a novel P2T-receptor antagonist AR-C69931 in a canine model. J Am Coll Cardiol. 2000;35(suppl): 281A–2.

42. Akers WS, Oh JJ, Oestreich JH, Ferraris S, et al. Pharmacokinetics and pharmacodynamics of a bolus and infusion of cangrelor: a direct, parenteral P2Y$_{12}$ receptor antagonist. J Clin Pharmacol. 2010;50: 27–35.

43. Harrington RA, Stone GW, McNulty S, White HD, Lincoff AM, Gibson CM, Pollack Jr CV, Montalescot G, Mahaffey KW, Kleiman NS, Goodman SG, Amine M, Angiolillo DJ, Becker RC, Chew DP, French WJ, Leisch F, Parikh KH, Skerjanec S, Bhatt DL. Platelet inhibition with cangrelor in patients undergoing PCI. N Engl J Med. 2009;361:2318–29.

44. Bhatt DL, Lincoff AM, Gibson CM, Stone GW, McNulty S, Montalescot G, Kleiman NS, Goodman SG, White HD, Mahaffey KW, Pollack Jr CV, Manoukian SV, Widimsky P, Chew DP, Cura F, Manukov I, Tousek F, Jafar MZ, Arneja J, Skerjanec S, Harrington RA, CHAMPION PLATFORM Investigators. Intravenous platelet blockade with cangrelor during PCI. N Engl J Med. 2009;361: 2330–41.

45. Bhatt DL, Stone GW, Mahaffey KW, Gibson CM, Steg PG, Hamm CW, Price MJ, Leonardi S, Gallup D, Bramucci E, Radke PW, Widimský P, Tousek F, Tauth J, Spriggs D, McLaurin BT, Angiolillo DJ, Généreux P, Liu T, Prats J, Todd M, Skerjanec S, White HD, Harrington RA, CHAMPION PHOENIX Investigators. Effect of platelet inhibition with cangrelor during PCI on ischemic events. N Engl J Med. 2013;368(14):1303–13.

46. Angiolillo DJ, Firstenberg MS, Price MJ, Tummala PE, Hutyra M, Welsby IJ, Voeltz MD, Chandna H, Ramaiah C, Brtko M, Cannon L, Dyke C, Liu T, Montalescot G, Manoukian SV, Prats J, Topol EJ. Bridging antiplatelet therapy with cangrelor in patients undergoing cardiac surgery: a randomized controlled trial. JAMA. 2012;307: 265–74.

47. Gretler DD, Conley PB, Andre P, et al. "First in human" experience with PRT060128, a new directacting, reversible, $P2Y_{12}$ inhibitor for IV and oral use. J Am Coll Cardiol. 2007;9 Suppl 2:326A.

48. Gurbel PA, Bliden KP, Antonino MJ, et al. The effect of elinogrel on high platelet reactivity during dual antiplatelet therapy and the relation to CYP2C19*2 genotype: first experience in patients. J Thromb Haemost. 2010;8:43–53.

49. Müller KA, Geisler T, Gawaz M. Elinogrel, an orally and intravenously available ADP-receptor antagonist. How does elinogrel affect a personalized antiplatelet therapy? Hamostaseologie. 2012; 32(3):191–4.

50. Berger JS, Roe MT, Gibson CM, Kilaru R, Green CL, Melton L, Blankenship JD, Metzger DC, Granger CB, Gretler DD, Grines CL, Huber K, Zeymer U, Buszman P, Harrington RA, Armstrong PW. Safety and feasibility of adjunctive antiplatelet therapy with intravenous elinogrel, a direct-acting and reversible $P2Y_{12}$ ADP-receptor antagonist, before primary percutaneous intervention in patients with ST-elevation myocardial infarction: the Early Rapid ReversAl of platelet thromboSis with intravenous Elinogrel before PCI to optimize reperfusion in acute Myocardial Infarction (ERASE MI) pilot trial. Am Heart J. 2009;158(6):998–1004.

51. Welsh RC, Rao SV, Zeymer U, Thompson VP, Huber K, Kochman J, McClure MW, Gretler DD, Bhatt DL, Gibson CM, Angiolillo DJ, Gurbel PA, Berdan LG, Paynter G, Leonardi S, Madan M, French WJ, Harrington RA, INNOVATE-PCI Investigators. A randomized, double-blind, active-controlled phase 2 trial to evaluate a novel selective and reversible intravenous and oral $P2Y_{12}$ inhibitor elinogrel versus clopidogrel in patients undergoing nonurgent percutaneous coronary intervention: the INNOVATE-PCI trial. Circ Cardiovasc Interv. 2012;5(3):336–46.

52. Zhao L, Bath PM, Fox S, May J, Judge H, Lösche W, Heptinstall S. The effects of GPIIb-IIIa antagonists and a combination of three other antiplatelet agents on platelet-leukocyte interactions. Curr Med Res Opin. 2003;19:178–86.
53. Roffi M, Chew DP, Mukherjee D, Bhatt DL, White JA, Moliterno DJ, Heeschen C, Hamm CW, Robbins MA, Kleiman NS, Théroux P, White HD, White HD, Topol EJ. Platelet glycoprotein IIb/IIIa inhibition in acute coronary syndromes. Gradient of benefit related to the revascularization strategy. Eur Heart J. 2002;23:1441–8.
54. Angiolillo DJ, Ueno M. Optimizing platelet inhibition in clopidogrel poor metabolizers: therapeutic options and practical considerations. J Am Coll Cardiol Cardiovasc Interv. 2011;4:411–4.

Chapter 3
Anticoagulation Therapy. Heparins, Factor II and Factor Xa Inhibitors

Ana Muñiz-Lozano, Fabiana Rollini, Francesco Franchi, and Dominick J. Angiolillo

Introduction and General Considerations

Atherosclerotic disease is a progressive and diffuse disease which may affect any arterial vasculature [1]. Coronary artery disease (CAD) starts in the late teens under the form of fatty streaks and progress with age, until atherosclerotic plaques are developed. Thrombotic complications of atherosclerotic plaques occur mostly following rupture, fissure or superficial endothelial cell erosion [2]. This leads to activation of the platelet cascade, characterized by adhesion, activation, and aggregation, as well as activation of the extrinsic pathway of the coagulation cascade which ultimately results in thrombin generation. Thrombus formation can be subclinical, and thus favor plaque progression, or clinical, and thus leading a clinical manifestation of an acute coronary syndrome (ACS) [1, 2]. Nonocclusive thrombi typically lead to a non-ST elevation ACS (NSTE-ACS) and occlusive thrombi to

A. Muñiz-Lozano, MD • F. Rollini, MD • F. Franchi, MD
D.J. Angiolillo, MD, PhD (✉)
Department of Cardiology,
University of Florida College of Medicine-Jacksonville,
655 West 8th Street, Jacksonville, FL 32209, USA
e-mail: dominick.angiolillo@jax.ufl.edu

P. Avanzas, P. Clemmensen (eds.), *Pharmacological Treatment*
of Acute Coronary Syndromes, Current Cardiovascular Therapy,
DOI 10.1007/978-1-4471-5424-2_3,
© Springer-Verlag London 2014

a ST-elevation myocardial infarction (STEMI) [1–3]. The absence or presence of cardiac biomarkers allows to differentiate NSTE-ACS patients into two categories: unstable angina (UA) or non-ST elevation myocardial infarction (NSTEMI). In the setting of percutaneous coronary interventions (PCI), plaque rupture is iatrogenically induced. Therefore, these patients are also exposed to the risk of intraprocedural thrombotic complications which warrant specific therapies.

The extensive procoagulant and prothrombotic actions of thrombin underlie its key role in the setting of ACS, given that it represents the last step of coagulation as it converts fibrinogen to clottable fibrin by releasing fibrinopeptides A and B [4]. Moreover, thrombin is also the most potent naturally occurring platelet agonist and therefore has been considered as a pharmacological target in order to prevent the formation of fibrin- and platelet-rich thrombi induced by thrombin. The mechanism of generation of acute platelet-rich thrombus and promoting vascular healing after arterial injury has been broadly described [5–10]. On the platelet surface, thrombin binds to its specific receptor on platelets ultimately leading to the expression of activated glycoprotein IIb/IIIa (GP IIb/IIIa) receptors. Via the GP IIb/IIIa receptor platelets are cross-link activated by ligands such as fibrinogen forming platelet aggregates. Moreover such platelet aggregates increase the surface area for the prothrombinase complex by providing a phospholipid membrane platform on which a complex of activated factors V and X and calcium ions can form contributing to thrombus formation [7] and amplifying thrombin generation. Thrombin becomes resistant to inactivation by the heparin/ antithrombin complex when bound to fibrin, fibrin degradation products or subendothelial matrix [8–10].

Given that this central role of thrombin in arterial thrombogenesis, therapeutic agents have been developed to target either thrombin or modulators of thrombin generation within the coagulation cascade (Fig. 3.1). These include a variety of agents available for parenteral administration, used in combination with antiplatelet therapies (discussed in details elsewhere in this book), used in ACS and PCI setting

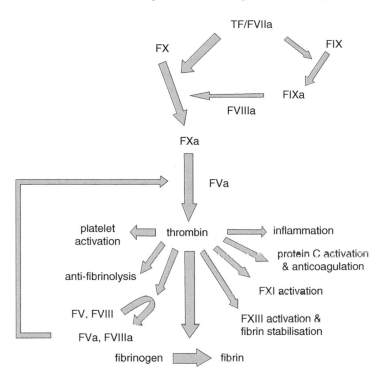

FIGURE 3.1   Central role of thrombin in thrombosis and haemostasis. Thrombin is a crucial enzyme that has numerous biological actions. Its main role regards the generation of fibrin by the excision of fibrinogen, but additionally it promotes platelet activation and aggregation by binding protease-activated receptors (PARs)-1 and −4 existing in platelets and multiple cell types exerts. Moreover, thrombin also intensifies clotting by activating coagulation factor (F) XI and the cofactors FV and FVIII into FVa and FVIIIa, respectively; and it stabilizes clots by activating FXIII. In addition, thrombin has pro-inflammatory actions and also exerts anti-fibrinolytic actions, given that it provides a molecular link between coagulation and inhibition of fibrinolysis by activating thrombin activatable fibrinolysis inhibitor (TAFI). Furthermore, thrombin promotes the activation of protein C and protein S, two natural vitamin K-dependent anticoagulant proteins that stop the coagulation cascade by blocking FVa and FVIIIa (Reproduced from De Caterina et al. [11])

which may be chosen depending on the level of ischemic and hemorrhagic risk of the patient as well as their planned early management (conservative vs. invasive). Indeed, not only the choice of therapy by also timing of administration and cessation are key determinant of short and long-term outcomes. Given that ACS patients persist with elevated thrombin levels following an ACS event, there also has been an emerging interest on adding oral anticoagulant therapy to standard antiplatelet regiment for long-term secondary prevention of ischemic event. In this chapter, we provide an overview of the basic principles of pharmacology, rationale for use, indications, contraindications, dosing considerations and side effects of currently available anticoagulant therapies are summarized and recent advances in the field provided.

Anticoagulant Therapy: Classification

The classification of anticoagulant agents is based primarily on the target coagulation enzyme which is inhibited. Most clinically available anticoagulant therapies block factor (F) II or thrombin and FX. Each class of inhibitors blocking a specific target can then be classified according to its mechanism of action to exert its inhibitory effects as direct or indirect, based on the need of a co-factor without which these agents would provide minimal or null effects (Fig. 3.2). Finally, anticoagulant therapies can be classified according to their route of administration (parenteral or oral).In the setting of ACS and PCI, parenteral agents are used and include a variety of thrombin inhibitors (direct and indirect). Anti-X inhibitors are also used in ACS patients, mostly medically managed, although to a lesser extent than thrombin inhibitors and currently only an indirect anti-X inhibitor for parenteral use is clinically available. These agents are described in details below.

Thrombin Inhibitors

Thrombin inhibitors can be classified into two broad categories according to the presence or absence of a plasma cofactor needed to exert its effects: indirect and direct thrombin inhibitors (DTIs). Details of these agents are described below.

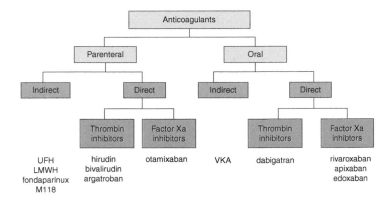

FIGURE 3.2 Currently available anticoagulants according their mode of action and route of administration (Reproduced from De Caterina et al. [11])

Indirect Thrombin Inhibitors

Indirect thrombin inhibitors include unfractionated heparin (UFH) and low-molecular weight heparin (LMWH), which in the absence of the cofactor antithrombin (AT), an endogenous inhibitor of several activated clotting factors have minimal or no intrinsic anticoagulant activity.

Unfractionated Heparin

Mechanism of Action and Pharmacokinetic/ Pharmacodynamic Profile

UFH is a highly sulfated glycosaminoglycan composed by a heterogeneous mixture of variable molecular weight polysaccharide molecules. The structure and the mechanism of action of heparin are described in Fig. 3.3. UFH is administrated through anintravenous (IV) or subcutaneous (SC) route because its polysaccharide chain is degraded in gastric acid. UFH should not be administrated intramuscularly because of the danger of hematoma generation. UFH is metabolized primarily by the liver (by heparinase to uroheparin, which has only small AT activity) and partially metabolized by the reticuloendothelial system [13].

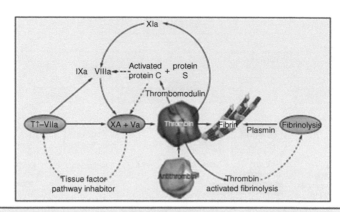

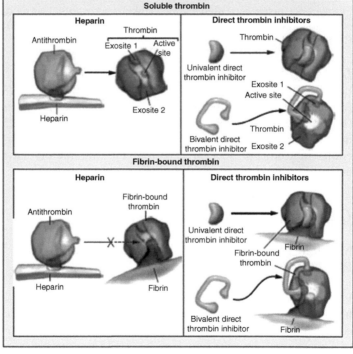

FIGURE 3.3 Mechanism of thrombin generation and action of direct thrombin inhibitors (DTIs) as compared with heparin. (**a**) Tissue-factor expression by endothelial cells and the activation of factors XI, IX, and VIII are crucial to formation of fibrin. During the coagulation cascade the molecule of thrombin is the cornerstone. Natural anticoagulant mechanisms regulate the formation of the clot limiting the hemostatic process to the location of the injury to the vessel. (**b**) The transformation of AT from a slow to a very fast thrombin inhibitor causes a conformational change by the binding of pentasaccharide to AT. A ternary complex (UFH:AT:thrombin), composed by AT and thrombin, joined by UFH longer chains (>18 saccharide units) acting as a bridge between both molecules, leads to a greater inhibition of thrombin compared with FXa. In this way, UFH fibrin formation and inhibits thrombin-induced activation of platelets, factor V, and factor VIII, thereby preventing thrombus propagation (Reproduced from Di Nisio M et al. [12])

After administering an IV bolus followed by continuous IV infusion, an immediate anticoagulant effect can be achieved, which underscores this route of administration in patients with ACS. SC administrations (10 % lower bioavailability than IV) delay 1 hour (h) the anticoagulant effect of UFH, achieving the peak plasma levels at 3 h [14, 15]. After entering in the bloodstream, the binding of UFH to a number of plasma proteins, endothelial cells, macrophages, and von Willebrand factor (vWF), takes places, reducing its anticoagulant activity, leading to heparin resistance, and inhibiting vWF-dependent platelet function [16–19] The variability of anticoagulant response, particularly in patients with thromboembolic disorders, and its complex pharmaco-kinetic (PK) profile, is caused by the heterogeneity of UFH properties [16]. Clearance of UFH takes place by a saturable depolymerization process produced by the binding of UFH to endothelial cells and macrophages [20, 21]. A non saturable renal clearance, a slower elimination pathway, occurs mostly with supraclinical doses of UFH [22].

The PK profile of UFH explains why the intensity and duration of anticoagulant response results nonlinear to therapeutic doses of UFH and increases excessively with cumulative dose. In line with this, an IV bolus of 100 U/kg increases the biological half-life of UFH from 30 min (after an IV bolus of 25 U/kg) to 60 min, and a bolus of 400 U/kg for 30–150 min [14, 22–24]. The anticoagulant effect of UFH lasts just a few hours after cessation of UFH due to the fast clearance. In fact, it is possible to reactivate the coagulation process and because of an increase of thrombin activity after cessation a phenomenon called "heparin rebound" may occur, despite concomitant aspirin treatment [25, 26]. Changing from IV to SC dosing before interruption of UFH could mitigate this effect [27, 28].

The heterogeneous binding properties to several cells and proteins confer UFH other biologic effects in addition to its anticoagulant effects, such as alteration of platelet function, an increase in vessel wall permeability, a suppression of smooth muscle cell proliferation. Inhibition of osteoblast formation and osteoclast activation has also been described by *in vitro* studies of UFH [28–35]. Clinically the most relevant non anticoagulant effect of UFH is its potential to induce immune-mediated platelet activation known as heparin-induced thrombocytopenia (HIT) [24, 36, 37].In comparison with LMWH,UFH causes more frequently thrombocytopenia (defined as a platelet count <100,000/μL or a 50 % reduction in baseline platelet count), with an approximate incidence of 0.3 %. The phenomenon of inadequate response to UFH is described by heparin resistance, demanding higher than usual doses of UFH to acquire the desired anticoagulant effect. More rapid clearance of UFH [38], increased heparin-binding proteins [17], AT deficiency, or increased factor VIII levels [39] can explain this phenomenon.

Indications

The benefit of UFH in the setting of ACS, particularly UA/NSTEMI, has been extensively demonstrated in many trials establishing it as a class IA therapy concomitantly with platelet inhibitors [40, 41]. Metaanalyses of six relatively small randomized, placebo-controlled trials with UFH for treatment of UA/NSTEMI have led to guideline recommendations for UFH use in ACS [42–48] (Table 3.1).

For STEMI patients undergoing PCI the use bivalirudin with or without prior treatment with UFH is considered preferable to UFH andglycoprotein IIb/IIIa inhibitors (GPI) [49, 50] (Table 3.2). However, during PCI or combined with fibrinolytic therapy in the setting of STEMI adjunctive anticoagulation with UFH has been also demonstrated in clinical trials, but the use of SC or IV UFH as an adjunct to streptokinase (SK) remains controversial. UFH is recommended in high-thrombotic-risk patients SK-treated [49, 50].

Dosages, Monitoring and Reversal

Based on evidence-based guideline recommendations and available clinical trial data [49, 50], initial dosing of UFH in patients with ACS should start with an IV weight-based bolus followed by continuous IV infusion [40]. At each institution, because of the laboratory variation, nomograms should be performed in order to reach activated partial thromboplastin time (aPTT) values in the target range, for many aPTT reagents [40, 49]. In a patient with ACS, UFH is usually initiated at time of clinical presentation. For UA/NSTEMI, an initial IV bolus of 60–70 U/kg (maximum 4,000 U) followed by continuous infusion of 12–15 U/kg/h (maximum 1,000 U/h is recommended) [40, 49]. For STEMI patients on non-SK fibrinolytic therapy regimens, the dosing of UFH is at the lower end of this range (Table 3.1) [51]. Given that higher aPTT responses to UFH have been related with older age, low body weight, and female sex, these factors should be particularly considered in dosing decisions. Also smoking and diabetes should be considered because have been associated with an attenuated response to UFH [52, 53]. Higher than usual doses of UFH to obtain the desired anticoagulant effect are needed when the phenomenon of inadequate response to UFH occurs because of a heparin resistance [17]. Higher doses of UFH, [54, 55] prolonged or repeated exposure, [56]

TABLE 3.1 Guidelines recommendations on anticoagulant therapy in unstable angina and non ST-elevation myocardial infarction patients

		Initial medical treatment	During PCI		After PCI
			Patient received initial medical treatment	Patient did not receive initial medical treatment	
2012 ACCF/AHA Guideline for the management of UA/NSTEMI* [40]	Bivalirudin	0.1 mg/kg bolus, 0.25 mg/kg/h infusion	0.5 mg/kg bolus, increase infusion to 1.75 mg/kg/h	0.75 mg/kg bolus, 1.75 mg/kg/h infusion	No additional treatment or continue infusion for up to 4 h
	Enoxaparin	LD of 30 mg IV bolus may be given MD = 1 mg/kg SC every 12 h; extend dosing interval to 1 mg/kg every 24 h if estimated creatinine clearance less than 30 ml/min	Last SC dose less than 8 h: 0.5–0.75 mg/kg no additional treatment Last SC dose greater than 8 h: 0.3 mg/kg IV bolus	IV bolus	No additional treatment
	Fondaparinux	2.5 mg SC once daily. Avoid for creatinine clearance less than 30 mL/min	50–60 U/kg IV bolus of UFH is recommended by the OASIS 5 Investigators	50–60 U/kg IV bolus of UFH is recommended by the OASIS 5 Investigators	No additional treatment
	Unfractionated heparin	LD of 60 U/kg (max 4,000 U) as IV bolus MD of IV infusion of 12 U/kg/h (max 1,000 U/h) to maintain aPTT at 1.5–2.0 times control (approximately 50–70 s)	IV GPI planned: target ACT 200 s No IV GPI planned: target ACT 250–300 s for HemoTec; 300–350 s for Hemochron	IV GPI planned: 60–70 U/kg No IV GPI planned: 100–140 U/kg	No additional treatment

2011 ESC Guideline for the management of UA/ NSTEMI** [11, 41]	Bivalirudin	If immediate invasive strategy is planned, bivalirudin without a GPI should be considered the anticoagulant of choice over UFH or enoxaparin, particularly in patients with a high risk of bleeding, provided that optimal DAPT with aspirin plus an ADP receptor blocker is given (Class I, LOE B) Bivalirudin plus provisional GPI are recommended as an alternative to UFH plus GPI in patients with an intended urgent or early invasive strategy, particularly in patients with a high risk of bleeding (Class I, LOE B)	Discontinuation of anticoagulation should be considered after an invasive procedure unless otherwise indicated (Class IIa, LOE C)
	Enoxaparin	For conservative or non-immediate invasive strategies 1 mg/kg twice daily is recommended when fondaparinux is not available (Class I, LOE B)	
	Fondaparinux	2.5 mg subcutaneously daily is preferred over other anticoagulants (Class I, LOE A) if planned: 1. A non-immediate invasive strategy or 2. A conservative strategy (treatment should be maintained until clinical discharge) (Class I, LOE A)	85 IU/kg IV bolus of UFH (adapted to ACT) or 60 IU in the case of concomitant use of GPI (Class I, LOE B)

(continued)

TABLE 3.1 (continued)

		During PCI		
	Initial medical treatment	Patient received initial medical treatment	Patient did not receive initial medical treatment	After PCI
Unfractionated heparin	For high-risk patients in whom an immediate invasive strategy is planned, UFH is preferred over LMWH or fondaparinux because of its shorter half-life and potential for complete reversal with protamine sulphate should bleeding occur (Class IIa B) For conservative or non-immediate invasive strategies if fondaparinux or enoxaparin are not available, UFH with a target aPTT of 50–70s or other LMWHs at the specific recommended doses are indicated (Class I, LOE C)	IV bolus under ACT guidance (ACT 250–350 s, or 200–250 s if a GPI is given) or weight-adjusted (usually 70–100 IU/kg, or 50–60 IU/kg) in combination with a GPI In patients with previous IV infusion of UFH: a further IV bolus of UFH adapted according to the ACT values and use of GPI		

LOE level of evidence, *ACT* activated clotting time, *aPTT* activated partial thromboplastin time, *GPI* glycoprotein IIb/IIIa receptor inhibitors, *LMWH* low molecular weight heparin, *PCI* percutaneous coronary intervention, *UFH* unfractionated heparin, *IU* international unit, *IV* intravenous, *SC* subcutaneous, *U* units, *UA/NSTEMI* unstable angina/non-ST-elevation myocardial infarction, *DAPT* dual antiplatelet therapy, *ADP* adenosine diphosphate

2012 ACCF/AHA Guideline for the management of UA/NSTEMI* [40]

- For conservatively managed patient who develops a need for PCI:

  (A) If fondaparinux was given for initial medical treatment an IV bolus of 50–60 U/kg of UFH is recommended (the safety of this drug combination is not well established).

  (B) If enoxaparin was the initial medical treatment additional IV enoxaparin is an acceptable option.

- For patients managed by an initial conservative strategy, enoxaparin and fondaparinux are more convenient because of their SC administration (compared with an IV infusion of UFH) and their lower association with heparin-induced thrombocytopenia (compared with UFH).

2011 ESC Guideline for the management of UA/NSTEMI** [11, 41]

- It is not recommended (Class III):

  – The use of SC UFH as an anticoagulation strategy, even as short-term bridging therapy (LOE B).

  – The use of a fixed aPTT target in seconds when using UFH for any therapeutic indication (LOE B).

  – The interchange of the various LMWH preparations (LOE B).

  – The crossover (switching) between heparins (UFH and LMWH) (LOE B).

  – The use of fondaparinux for prevention or treatment of thrombosis during pregnancy, unless the patient has a history of HIT (LOE B).

  – The use of LMWH as alternatives to heparin in patients with suspected or established HIT (LOE A).

(continued)

- In patients with chronic kidney disease:
  - Moderate (CrCl 30–60 ml/min): reducing enoxaparin to 75 % of the usual dose (Class IIa, LOE B).
  - Severe or end-stage (CrCl ≤15–30 ml/min):
    - UFH over LMWH and over fondaparinux (Class I A).
    - The IV infusion dose of bivalirudin should be reduced from 1.75 to 1 mg/kg/h
  - Haemodialysis: The IV infusion dose of bivalirudin should be reduced from 1.75 to 0.25 mg/kg/h
- Regarding monitoring:
  - The therapeutic range for UFH should be adapted to the aPTT reagent used (Class IIa, LOE B).
  - The anticoagulant activity of LMWH or fondaparinux can be measured with anti-FXa assays, using the appropriate reference calibrator (Class I, LOE B).

TABLE 3.2 Guidelines recommendations on anticoagulant therapy in ST-elevation myocardial infarction patients

	Undergoing primary percutaneous coronary intervention	Receiving fibrinolytic therapy

2013 ACCF/ AHA guideline for the management of STEMI [49]	**UFH**: Class I LOE C
	
	With GPI planned: 50- to 70-U/kg IV bolus to achieve therapeutic ACT
	With no GPI planned: 70- to 100-U/kg bolus to achieve therapeutic ACT.
	
	Bivalirudin: Class I LOE B
	0.75-mg/kg IV bolus, then 1.75-mg/kg/h infusion with or without prior treatment with UFH. An additional bolus of 0.3 mg/kg can be given if needed.
	Reduce infusion to 1 mg/kg/h with estimated CrCl <30 mL/min. [Class I LOE B]
	Preferred over UFH with GPI in patients at high risk of bleeding. [Class IIa LOE B]
	Preferred over UFH with GPI in patients at high risk of bleeding. [Class IIa LOE B]
		UFH:
		To support reperfusion
		  Weight-based IV bolus and infusion adjusted to obtain aPTT of 1.5–2.0 times control for 48 h or until revascularization.
		  IV bolus of 50 U/kg (maximum 4,000 U) followed by an infusion of 12 U/kg/h (maximum 1,000 U) initially, adjusted to maintain aPTT at 1.5–2.0 times control (approximately 50–70 s) for 48 h or until revascularization.
		To Support PCI After Fibrinolytic Therapy
		  Continue UFH through PCI, administering additional IV boluses as needed to maintain therapeutic ACT depending on use of GPI.
		  ACT recommended without GPI:
		    250–300 s (HemoTec device) or
		    300–350 s (Hemochron device).
		  [Class I LOE C]
		
		Bivalirudin: Not recommended.

(continued)

TABLE 3.2 (continued)

Undergoing primary percutaneous coronary intervention	Receiving fibrinolytic therapy

Enoxaparin: Not recommended.	**Enoxaparin:**
	To support reperfusion [Class I LOE A]
	<75 years: 30 mg IV bolus, followed in 15 min by 1 mg/kg SC every 12 h (max. 100 mg for the first 2 doses).
	≥75 years: no bolus, 0.75 mg/kg SC every 12 h (maximum 75 mg for the first 2 doses).
	CrCl <30 mL/min: 1 mg/kg SC every 24 h.
	Duration: For the index hospitalization, up to 8 days or until revascularization.
	To Support PCI After Fibrinolytic Therapy
	Continue enoxaparin through PCI:
	  No additional drug if last dose within previous 8 h
	  0.3-mg/kg IV bolus if last dose 8–12 h earlier.
	[Class I LOE B]

Fondaparinux: Class III LOE B Not recommended as sole anticoagulant for primary PCI	**Fondaparinux:** To support reperfusion [Class I LOE B] Initial dose 2.5 mg IV, then 2.5 mg SC daily starting the following day, for the index hospitalization up to 8 days or until revascularization. Contraindicated if CrCl <30 mL/min. To Support PCI After Fibrinolytic Therapy Not recommended as sole anticoagulant for primary PCI [Class III LOE C]

2012 ESC Guidelines for the management of AMI in patients presenting with ST-segment elevation [50]	An injectable anticoagulant must be used in primary PCI. Class I LOE C. **Bivalirudin**: Class I LOE B With GPI restricted to bailout is recommended over UFH and a GPI. 0.75 mg/kg IV bolus followed by IV infusion of 1.75 mg/kg/h for up to 4 h after the procedure as clinically warranted. After cessation of the 1.75 mg/kg/h infusion, a reduced infusion dose of 0.25 mg/kg/h may be continued for 4–12 h as clinically necessary. **Enoxaparin**: with or without routine GPI. Class IIb LOE B May be preferred over UFH. 0.5 mg/kg IV bolus.	**Bivalirudin**: Not recommended. **Enoxaparin**: Preferred over UFH for patients <75 years of age and have an estimated CrCl >30 ml/min [Class IIa LOE B]. <75 years: 30 mg IV bolus followed 15 min later by 1 mg/kg SC every 12 h until hospital discharge for a maximum of 8 days (the first two doses should not exceed 100 mg). >75 years: no IV bolus; start with first SC dose of 0.75 mg/kg with a maximum of 75 mg for the first two SC doses. In patients with CrCl <30 mL/min, regardless of age, the SC doses are given once every 24 h.

(continued)

TABLE 3.2 (continued)

Undergoing primary percutaneous coronary intervention	Receiving fibrinolytic therapy
UFH: with or without routine GPI. Class I LOE C Must be used in patients not receiving bivalirudin or enoxaparin. 70–100 U/kg IV bolus when no GPI is planned. 50–60 U/kg IV bolus with GPI.	**UFH**: Agent of choice for patients >75 years of age or with a CrCl <30 ml/min. [Class I LOE B] 60 U/kg IV bolus with a maximum of 4,000 U followed by an IV infusion of 12 U/kg with a maximum of 1,000 U/h for 24-48 h. Target aPTT: 50–70 s or 1.5–2.0 times that of control to be monitored at 3, 6, 12 and 24 h.
Fondaparinux: Class III LOE B Not recommended for primary PCI.	**Fondaparinux**: As effective and safe as UFH, provided CrCl is >30 ml/min. [Class IIa LOE B] 2.5 mg IV bolus followed by a SC dose of 2.5 mg once daily up to 8 days or hospital discharge.

ACC American College of Cardiology Foundation/American Heart Association, *ESC* European Society of Cardiology, *STEMI* ST-elevation myocardial infarction, *AMI* acute myocardial infarction, *UFH* unfractionated heparin, *GPI* glycoprotein IIb/IIIa inhibitor, *LOE* level of evidence, *IV* intravenous, *PCI* percutaneous coronary intervention, *CrCl* creatinine clearance and concomitant use of fibrinolytic [57–59] or GPI [60] have been associated with an increase of the hemorrhagic and non-hemorrhagic complications. During UFH infusion platelet count and hemoglobin should be measured at least once a day. More than a 20 % of patients could have a mild, clinically insignificant drop in their platelet count (above 100,000/µL). All UFH therapy (included IV flush) should be immediately interrupted if there is a drop in platelet count (suspecting HIT). Moreover a screening for anti–platelet factor-4 antibodies, followed by the more definitive serotonin release assay, is also required [56, 61, 62]. Reversal of UFH effects can be achieved with protamine, a small arginine-rich (e.g. cationic) nuclear protein purified from fish sperm. An IV bolus of 1 mg of protamine could be used to rapidly neutralize 100 U of UFH, reversing its anticoagulant effect [63, 64].

In the setting of PCI, the recommended dosage of IV UFH depends on prior exposure to anticoagulant therapy [65] (Table 3.2). In patients who have received prior anticoagulant therapy, if IV GPI are planned, UFH should be added as needed (e.g., 2,000–5,000 U) to achieve an ACT of 200–250 s. If IV GPI are not planned, the additional UFH should aim to achieve an ACT of 250–300 s for HemoTec, 300–350 s for Hemochron. Without prior anticoagulant therapy, if IV GPI are planned, a 50–70 U/kg bolus should be administrated to achieve an ACT of 200–250 s. However, if IV GPI are not planned, the bolus dose may be 70–100 U/kg to achieve target ACT of 250–300 s for HemoTec, 300–350 s for Hemochron. Full-dose anticoagulation is no longer used after successful PCI procedures [65].

Side Effects and Contraindications

Bleeding is the main side effect related with the use of IV UFH, but recent trials demonstrated that this is <3 % [66]. However, higher heparin dosages, concomitant use of anti-platelet drugs or oral anticoagulant, and increasing age (>70 years) increases the bleeding risk [66]. As stated above, the development of HIT (usually between 5 and 15 days after the initiation of UFH) is another important problem associated with heparin therapy. Patients who have a previous exposition to heparin may have a more rapid onset [36, 37, 61].An alternative antithrombin drug must be chosen in the setting of HIT. The development of osteoporosis and rare allergic reactions less commonly have been described with long-term use of heparin.

Low-Molecular-Weight Heparin

Mechanism of Action and Pharmacokinetic/ Pharmacodynamic Profile

Because of the many known limitations associated with the use of UFH (nonspecific binding, the production of antiheparin antibodies that may induce thrombocytopenia, continuous IV infusion, and the necessity for frequent monitoring), LMWHs, potent inhibitors of both thrombin (anti-IIa effects) and FXa have been developed [55]. These heparins do not require monitoring due to their more rapid and predictable absorption, anticoagulant response and greater than 90 % bioavailability [67]. Anti-Xa levels peak 3–5 h after a SC dose of LMWH [68, 69]. Fewer platelet agonist effects less often associated with HIT also characterize LMWHs. After 3–6 h following a SC dose a renal elimination (largely dose-independent) takes place, leading to prolonged anti-Xa effect and linear accumulation of anti-Xa activity in patients with a creatinine clearance (CrCl) <30 ml/min [70–72]. The anticoagulant effect of LMWHs can be measured via anti-FXa levels, with a target peak anti-Xa level 0.6–1.0 U/mL derived from studies of venous thromboembolism treatment [73, 74].

Depolymerization of the polysaccharide chains of UFH originates LMWHs, producing fragments ranging from 2,000 to 10,000 Da [68, 69, 75]. The unique pentasaccharide sequence needed to bind to AT is contained by these shorter chain lengths, that are too short (<18 saccharides) to form the ternary complex crosslinking AT and thrombin. Consequently, the primary effect of LMWHs is limited to AT-dependent FXa inhibition. LMWHs result in a FXa:thrombin inhibition ratio ranging from 2 to 4:1, in comparison to UFH where the ratio of FXa:thrombin inhibition is 1:1 [76]. Also compared to UFH, LMWHs have a more favorable and predictable pharmacokinetic profile because of its reduced binding to plasma proteins and cells [68].

Enoxaparin is the most studied and developed LMWH preparation in clinical trials of UA/NSTEMI, STEMI and PCI. The main difference among LMWHs is their molecular weight and therefore the relative anti-Xa:anti IIa ratio. Enoxaparin has a mean molecular weight of 4,200 Da with anti-Xa:anti-IIa ratio of 3.8; dalteparin with a mean molecular weight of 6,000 Da has an anti-Xa: anti-IIa ratio of 2.7 [69]. The preferential binding ratio to FXa over thrombin, less plasma protein binding, attenuated platelet activation, lower risk of HIT, and reduced binding to osteoblasts are the theoretical pharmacologic advantages of LMWH over UFH [35, 69, 77–79].

In the majority of clinical settings routine monitoring of anti-FXa levels is not necessary due to the predictable anticoagulant response to LMWHs. The Thrombolysis in Myocardial Infarction 11A (TIMI 11A) trial assessed the PK and pharmacodynamic (PD) properties of enoxaparin including an enoxaparin clearance of 0.733 L/h, a distribution volume of 5.24 L, and an elimination half-life of 5 h [80]. Enoxaparin clearance modeled and predicted hemorrhagic complications and was significantly related to patient weight and CrCl. A 27 % decrease in enoxaparin clearance was correlated with CrCl <30 mL/min, causing a 3.8-fold increased risk of major hemorrhage [81]. In patients with CrCl <30 mL/min, the dose of enoxaparin needs to be adjusted and reduced in half (e.g. 1 mg/kg/day). Age, female sex, lower body weight, reduced renal function, and interventional procedures can increase the risk of bleeding with LMWH which is highly dose-related [80].

The probability of LMWHs to origin anti–platelet factor-4 antibody formation is about three times lower than UFH [56,

82] and produces less frequently HIT in patients who have anti-platelet factor-4 antibodies, although LMWHs are similarly reactive as UFH in activation assays of washed platelets using serum from HIT patients [56, 83]. Also osteopenic effect is lower compared with UFH [84]. Protamine sulfate (1 mg per each 1 mg of enoxaparin within 8 h) may be used to neutralize the anti-IIa effect of LMWH when hemorrhagic complications, but it is variable and uncertain the grade to which the anti-Xa activity of LMWH is neutralized by protamine [85].

Indications

The safety and efficacy of LMWHs has been demonstrated in patients with UA/NSTEMI and STEMI, and also in patients undergoing PCI [40, 49, 86]. LMWH with UFH have been directly compared in 9 randomized trials [87–95] in UA/NSTEMI patients. No significant differences in death or MI were observed in patients treated with LMWH compared with UFH in two studies using dalteparin [87, 88] and one with nadroparin [89]. Enoxaparin's greater anti-Xa-to-anti-IIa ratio when compared with dalteparin, and the extension of its antithrombotic actions to include inhibition of platelet aggregation by blocking the release of vWF could be the reasons of the greater severity of the disease in the patients enrolled in the reported studies [96].

A meta-analysis by Petersen et al. [97] that pooled the data from six trials evaluating 21,946UA/NSTEMI patients randomized to enoxaparin or UFH, showed significant reductions in the combined endpoint of death/MI by 30 days favoring enoxaparin over UFH, particularly in patients who had not received any antithrombin before randomization [97]. There were no significant differences in major bleeding or blood transfusion within the first week of therapy.

The largest and most recent trial comparing enoxaparin to UFH, randomized 10,027 high-risk patients with UA/NSTEMI undergoing an early invasive strategy using guideline recommended aspirin, clopidogrel and GPI [90]. The primary composite end point of death or MI at 30 days, was no different between enoxaparin and UFH (14 % vs. 14.5 %; OR 0.96; 95 % CI, 0.86–1.06). Enoxaparin compared to UFH produced significantly higher TIMI major bleeding (P = 0.008). Anticoagulant switching effects due to pre-randomization anticoagulant use and time- rather than ACT-guided sheath removal in the enoxaparin arm were potential causes of the increased bleeding with enoxaparin [90]. Enoxaparin, but not the other LMWHs, is preferred over UFH for the medical management of UA/NSTEMI in the ACC/AHA guidelines [40]. The greatest benefit is described in patients with elevated troponin values.

As adjunctive pharmacotherapy for STEMI patients receiving fibrinolytic therapy, the safety and efficacy of enoxaparin versus UFH has been assessed in 2 trials. Added to fibrinolytic therapy, enoxaparin diminished the risk of in-hospital reinfarction or refractory ischemia compared to UFH, but at the expense of an increased the rate of intra-cranial hemorrhage (ICH) among patients over the age of 75 [49, 98, 99].

STEMI patients receiving thrombolytic therapy to enoxaparin or UFH for at least 48 h were randomized in the Enoxaparin and Thrombolysis Reperfusion for Acute Myocardial Infarction-TIMI 25 (ExTRACT TIMI 25) trial (n = 20,506) [51]. Patients with impaired renal function defined (CrCl <30 mL/min) received a reduced dose of enoxaparin (1 mg/kg SC q.d.) and also patients older than 75 did not receive bolus of enoxaparin and receive a lower SC dose of 0.75 mg/kg b.i.d). The risk of death and reinfarction at 30 days associated with enoxaparin compared with UFH was significantly reduced (p = 0.001). Enoxaparin was associated with a significant increase of TIMI major bleeding compared with UFH (2.1 % vs. 1.4 %; P < 0.001). In conclusion, the type of fibrinolytic agent and the age of the patient did not affect the net clinical benefit (absence of death, non-fatal infarction, or ICH) which favored enoxaparin (10.1 % vs. 12.2 %; P < 0.001) [100, 101].

Dosages

UA/NSTEMI patients should receive anticoagulant therapy in addition to antiplatelet therapy as soon as possible after clinical presentation [40, 49] (Table 3.1). Enoxaparin (1 mg/kg SC b.i.d) has demonstrated to be effective for patients in whom an invasive or conservative strategy is selected. As previously mentioned, it is particularly important to adjust the dose of enoxaparin in patients with renal insufficiency (CrCl <30 mL/min), reducing it to 1.0 mg/kg SC daily. LMWH should be continued without loading of UFH if it has been started upstream.

Numerous routes of administration of LMWH can be used in the setting of a PCI: (a) the first dosing regimen option is 1 mg/kg SC b.i.d.; the last dose of SC LMWH has to be administered within 8 h of the procedure and it is also important to warrant that at least 2 SC doses of LMWH are given before the procedure to ensure balanced state; (b) a 0.3 mg/kg bolus of IV enoxaparin is recommended at the time of PCI if the last dose of enoxaparin was given 8–12 h before PCI, (c) another dosing regimen option at the time of PCI is 1 mg/kg enoxaparin IV (if no GPIis used) or 0.75 mg/kg (if a GPI is used) [40, 49]. The STEEPLE (SafeTy and Efficacy of Enoxaparin in PCI patients, an internationaL randomized Evaluation) study found safe the IV dose of 0.5 mg/kg for elective PCI [102].

In the setting of patients with STEMI treated with fibrinolysis if renal function is preserved (<2.5 mg/dL [220 µmol/L] in male patients and <2.0 mg/dL [175 µmol/L] in female patients), we recommend the use of enoxaparin over UFH, continued up to 8 days (Class IIa, LOE B). The recommended dosing for enoxaparin depends on the age: 30-mg IV bolus followed by 1 mg/kg SC q12 h (maximum of 100 mg for the first two SC doses) for <75 years; and no IV bolus, 0.75 mg/kg SC q12 h (maximum of 75 mg for the first two SC doses) for age >75 years. Enoxaparin should be given before fibrinolytic administration. The continuation of enoxaparin therapy after discharge has not be demonstrated to be beneficial [49], and for this reason enoxaparin regimen uses to be maintained during hospitalization or until day 8 (whatever come first). Regardless of age, if the CrCl is <30 mL/min the dosage of 1 mg/kg subcutaneously every 24 h may be used.

For patients with STEMI undergoing PCI after receiving fibrinolytic therapy with enoxaparin, if the last SC dose was given within the prior 8 h, no additional enoxaparin should be administered; if the last SC dose was given between 8 and 12 h earlier, enoxaparin 0.3 mg/kg IV should be administered (Class I, LOE B) (Table 3.2). These recommendations are based on the analysis of patients who underwent PCI in the ExTRACT TIMI 25 trial [103] as well as on the Enoxaparin as adjunctive antithrombin therapy for ST-elevation myocardial infarction: results of the ENTIRE-TIMI 23 trial [104]. This trial demonstrated that enoxaparin was associated with similar TIMI 3 flow rates as UFH at an early time point, with similar risk of major hemorrhage and greater benefit over UFH regarding to ischemic events through 30 days (P = 0.005) [104].

Side Effects and Contraindications

Patients with contraindications to anticoagulant therapy such as active bleeding, significant thrombocytopenia, recent neurosurgery, ICH, or ocular surgery should not receive LMWH. Patients with bleeding diathesis, brain metastases, recent major trauma, endocarditis, and severe hypertension required to be treated with particular caution. Less major bleeding compared with UFH has been associated with enoxaparin in acute venous thromboembolism. In the setting of ACS, neither UFH nor LMWH are associated with an increase in major bleeding, but in ischemic stroke the both agents are associated with an increase in major bleeding [105]. Hemorrhagic complications could occur due to LMWH, particularly in patients with renal dysfunction (who should receive an adjusted dose of enoxaparin). To neutralize the anti-IIa effect of LMWH, protamine sulfate may be administered, although the degree of neutralization of the anti-Xa activity of LMWH is variable and uncertain. In patients with documented or suspected HIT,LMWH are not recommended for use because they can induce it.

Direct Thrombin Inhibitors

The direct thrombin inhibitors (DTIs) bind to thrombin and inhibit its capacity to transform fibrinogen to fibrin, to intensify its own generation through activation of FV, FVIII, and FIX, and to function as a potent platelet agonist [106]. Importantly, DTIs not only block free thrombin, but also inhibit thrombin bound to fibrin in contrast to indirect thrombin inhibitors [12, 107–109] (Fig. 3.3). These properties are indeed important and provide a rationale for their clinical use in the setting of ACS and PCI. The anticoagulant effect of DTIs in healthy volunteers can be reversed by recombinant factor VIIa, although the short half-life of these agents normally avoids the necessity for active reversal [110]. Three DTI's are approved for clinical use (lepirudin, argatroban, and bivalirudin) and described below.

Hirudin (lepirudin)

Mechanism of Action and Pharmacokinetic/ Pharmacodynamic Profile

Hirudin is among the most potent of the natural thrombin inhibitors. It is a 65-amino acid polypeptide located in the salivary glands of the leech *Hirudo medicinalis*. Lepirudin is a recombinant form of hirudin that irreversibly inhibits thrombin [111]. Several biochemical and molecular biological techniques have been used to study the specific nature of the hirudin-thrombin interaction. The thrombin time (TT) and the aPTT are the most frequently used measures for the anticoagulant activity of hirudin. Bleeding time is not significantly altered by hirudin which does not have direct effects on platelet aggregation or secretion.

Indications

In UA/NSTEMI a single dose of UFH with a single dose of hirudin were compared in both the TIMI-9 and the Global Utilization of Strategies to Open Occluded Coronary Arteries (GUSTO) II trials [57, 58]. Both trials used high doses of hirudin (0.6 mg/kg bolus followed by 0.2 mg/kg/h) and weight-adjusted heparin. An unacceptably high rate of ICH in both treatment arms forced to terminate prematurely both trials. Using lower doses of both hirudin (0.1 mg/kg bolus followed by 0.1 mg/kg/h) and heparin (not weight adjusted), both trials were continued as TIMI-9b [57] and GUSTO IIb [59]. The TIMI-9b trial showed similar efficacy of heparin and hirudin as adjunctive therapies for SK or t-PA in individuals with acute Q-wave MI without differences in bleeding [57]. The GUSTO IIb trial showed a marginally significant benefit of hirudin over heparin early after infarction in individuals with both Q wave and non–Q-wave MI, which lessened over time [59]. Additionally, results from the Organisation to Assess Strategies for Ischemic Syndromes (OASIS-2) trial showed that recombinant hirudin may be useful when compared with heparin in preventing cardiovascular death, MI, and refractory angina with an acceptable safety profile in patients who have UA/NSTEMI and who receive aspirin [112]. This study ($n = 10,141$) randomized patients to receive UFH or hirudin (0.4 mg/kg bolus, 0.15 mg/kg/h infusion) for 72 h. This study demonstrated a nonsignificant difference between hirudin and UFH in the primary outcome of cardiovascular death or MI at 7 days: 3.6 % vs.4.2 % had experienced cardiovascular death or new MI ($P = 0.077$). However, hirudin was associated with a significantly increased risk of major, but not life-threatening, bleeding [112].

A pooled analysis of the OASIS, GUSTO (Global Utilization of Streptokinase and Tissue Plasminogen Activator for Occluded Arteries)-2B, and TIMI-9B trials showed superiority of hirudin compared with UFH for the prevention of death or MI at 30–35 days [112]. However, the only approved clinical application for this agent is in the treatment of HIT recombinant hirudin (lepirudin). Because of a reduced risk for new thromboembolic complications, lepirudin-treated patients had consistently lower incidences of combined endpoints primarily when compared with historical controls [12].

Dosage

The dosage of IV hirudin is 0.15 mg/kg/h infusion with or without 0.4 mg/kg initial bolus [113]. Monitoring is required and it has a narrow therapeutic window. During treatment with lepirudin, aPTT ratios of 1.5:2.5 produce optimal clinical efficacy with a moderate risk for bleeding, aPTT ratios lower than 1.5 are subtherapeutic, and aPTT levels greater than 2.5 are associated with high bleeding risk. The plasma half-life of hirudins is 60 min following IV injection [114]. Renal clearance is the predominant way of elimination of this drug. Adjustment of dose of lepirudin is recommended for patients with severe renal impairment (<30 ml/min) reducing the dose by a factor of six compared with that given to patients with normal renal function. Monitoring of aPTT should be necessary to further adjust if it exceeds two times baseline. In moderate (CrCl 31–60 ml/min) and mild renal impairment (CrCl 61–90 ml/min) adjustment is not recommended initially but if peak aPTT exceeds two times baseline it is necessary to reduce the dose by half [114].

Side Effects and Contraindications

In settings where anticoagulation is contraindicated hirudin should not be used. In the setting of concomitant anticoagulation or platelet inhibitors, the risk of bleeding with hirudin is increased. In patients with renal dysfunction hirudin should not be used (given that it is renally cleared). Antibody formation to hirudin can be induced for this agent in up to 40 % of patients, presenting anaphylaxis after a re-exposure [113].

Argatroban

Mechanism of Action and Pharmacokinetic/ Pharmacodynamic Profile

Argatroban or (2R,4R) 4-methyl-[N2-(3-methyl-1,2,3,4-tetrahydro-8-quinolinyl) sulfonyl]-2-piperidine carboxylic acid is a small-molecule with potent direct competitive thrombin inhibiting effects [12]. This drug is a synthetic N2-substituted arginine derivative that binds to the catalytic site of thrombin with high affinity. Itbinds noncovalently and rapidly to both clot-bound and soluble thrombin, forming in that way a reversible complex [115, 116]. Argatroban is metabolized via the cytochrome P450 3A4 pathway in the liver with a half-life of 45 min. Rapid restoration of normal hemostasis on cessation of therapy is allowed by the reversible binding of the agent. Argatroban has a predictable dose response that correlates with changes in anticoagulant parameters.

Indications

The use of argatroban has been evaluated primarily as adjunctive therapy with fibrinolytics, in the treatment of HIT, or in patients undergoing PCI [40, 49]. At present there are still limited data with argatroban and it is approved only for use in HIT [117].

Dosages

Argatroban is administered in individuals with unstable angina at a dose of 0.5–5.0 μg/kg/min for 4 h. Dose adjustment with renal impairment is unnecessary, but in patients with renal failure it should be used with caution [118].

Side Effects and Contraindications

Argatroban should not be used in patients who have contraindications to anticoagulant therapy. Argatroban metabolism occurs in the liver. The maximum concentration and half-life of argatroban are increased approximately two- to threefold and clearance is one fourth in patients with hepatic impairment compared with healthy volunteers.

Bivalirudin

Mechanism of Action and Pharmacokinetic/ Pharmacodynamic Profile

Bivalirudin is a 20-amino acid polypeptide and is a synthetic version of hirudin [119]. Its amino-terminal D-Phe-Pro-Arg-Pro domain, which interacts with active site of thrombin, is linked via 4 Gly residues to adodecapeptide analogue of the carboxy-terminal of hirudin (thrombinexosite) [120] (Fig. 3.3). Bivalirudin forms a 1:1 stoichiometric complex with thrombin, but once bound, the amino terminal of bivalirudin is cleaved by thrombin, thereby restoring thrombin activity [121].

The half-life of bivalirudin is 25 min [122]. Its clearance is mediated by proteolysis, hepatic metabolism, and renal excretion [123]. Severe renal impairment prolongs the half-life of bivalirudin, and dose adjustment is required for dialysis [124]. Bivalirudin is not immunogenic, in contrast to hirudin, although antibodies against hirudin can cross-react with bivalirudin, the clinical consequences of which are unknown [113].

Indications and Dosage

The use of bivalirudin is supported by wide clinical trial experience. These include supstream treatment in patients with UA/NSTEMI [125, 126],across the spectrum of patients of patients undergoing PCI, including patients with STEMI undergoing primary PCI as an alternative to UFH plus GPI [127], in patients undergoing CABG [128], and in HIT [129]. The recommended dose in PCI is a bolus of 0.75 mg/kg followed by an infusion of 1.75 mg/kg/h for up to 4 h after the procedure as clinically warranted. After cessation of the 1.75 mg/kg/h infusion, a reduced infusion dose of 0.25 mg/kg/h may be continued for 4–12 h as clinically necessary.

Evidence for Use: UA/NSTEMI

Bivalirudin and UFH were compared in the Randomized Evaluation in Percutaneous Coronary Intervention Linking Angiomax to Reduced Clinical Events 2(REPLACE-2) study [130]. This trial (n = 6,010) enrolled patients undergoing urgent or elective PCI who were randomized to receive bivalirudin with provisional GPI or UFH with planned GPI. The study demonstrated the noninferiority of bivalirudin compared to UFH plus GPI regarding ischemic end point sand showed also a significant association with less major and minor bleeding [130].

In the Acute Catheterization and Urgent Intervention Triage Strategy (ACUITY) study, patients with UA/NSTEMI (n = 13,189) were randomized to one of three antithrombotic regimens: UFH or enoxaparin plus GPI, bivalirudin plus GPI, or bivalirudin alone [125]. Compared with UFH plus a GPI, bivalirudin plus a GPI, was associated with noninferior 30-day rates of the composite ischemia end point (7.7 and 7.3 %, respectively), major bleeding (5.3 and 5.7 %), and the net clinical outcome end point (11.8 and 11.7 %). Compared with UFH plus a GPI, bivalirudin alone was associated with a noninferior rate of the composite ischemia end point (7.8 and 7.3 %, respectively; P = 0.32) and significantly reduced rates of major bleeding (3.0 % vs. 5.7 %; P < 0.001) and the net clinical outcome end point (10.1 % vs. 11.7 %; P = 0.02). Essentially, compared with UFH bivalirudin in addition to GPI presented similar rates of ischemia and bleeding, but bivalirudin alone was also associated with significantly lower rates of bleeding [125].

However, the ACUITY trial presented some important limitations that need to be addressed: first, not all patients were pretreated with clopidogrel (and used inconsistent dosing) and two thirds of them were already receiving some anticoagulant before randomization and, with the resultant variability among the treatments before and during the study. Moreover the election of type of GPI and UFH/LMWH was left at the discretion of physician. Lastly, the ACUITY trial has been also criticized because of its quite liberal definition of bleeding, particularly concerning the definition of major bleeding [125].

The Intracoronary Stenting and Antithrombotic Regimen: Rapid Early Action for Coronary Treatment 4 (ISAR REACT 4) trial [126] was a double-blind randomized trial which design tried to overcome the aforementioned limitations of the ACUITY trial. The same GPI (abciximab) was used and all patients received a 600-mg-clopidogrel pretreatment. In addition, less liberal definitions of major bleeding were considered (presence of intracranial, intraocular, or retroperitoneal hemorrhage; a decrease in the hemoglobin level of > 40 g/L plus either overt bleeding or the need for transfusion of 2 or more units of packed red cells or whole blood). Specifically, the ISAR REACT 4 trial compared abciximab and heparin versus bivalirudin in NSTEMI patients undergoing PCI (n = 1,721) showing that such regimen compared to bivalirudin increased the risk of bleeding in NSTEMI patients undergoing PCI (P = 0.02) and failed to decrease the rate of ischemic events (P = 0.76) [126]. Current guidelines for UA/NSTEMI recommend to omit administration of an IV GPI if bivalirudin is selected as the anticoagulant and at least 300 mg of cvs. lopidogrel was administered at least 6 h earlier than planned catheterization or PCI (Class IIa, LOE B) [40, 65] (Table 3.1).

Evidence for Use: STEMI

In the Harmonizing Outcomes with Revascularization and Stents in Acute Myocardial Infarctions (HORIZONS-AMI) trial, [127] STEMI patients (n = 3,602) who presented within 12 h after onset of symptoms were randomized to UFH plus

GPI or to treatment with bivalirudin alone for primary PCI. At 30 days, compared with UFH plus GPI, bivalirudin alone demonstrated lower rates of death (P = 0.047) and major bleeding (P < 0.001), leading to a significantly lower rate of net adverse clinical events (P = 0.005). The rates of cardiac mortality (P = 0.005) and all-cause mortality (P = 0.037) were significantly lower in the bivalirudin alone treatment group after 1 year (p = 0.001) [131] and 3 years (P = 0.03) [132]. Regarding stent thrombosis (ST), the study found that within the first 24 h ST occurred more commonly in patients on bivalirudin compared with those assigned to heparin plus a GPI [127]. Nevertheless, between 24 h and 1 year, ST was more frequent in the heparin plus GPI group than in the bivalirudin group (46 vs. 36 ST events, respectively). Thus, at the end of the 1-year follow-up, the rate of ST was similar in the two groups (3.1 % vs. 3.5 %, respectively, P = 0.53) [131]. However, the hazard ratio for death within the first month was greater after major bleeding than after reinfarction or ST [127]. In a post-hoc analysis, mortality and major bleeding were shown to be significantly higher after in-hospital ST compared with out-of-hospital ST (p < 0.01 for both events). Randomization to UFH plus GPI (vs. bivalirudin) was additionally correlated with increased mortality after ST [133].

Another post-hoc analysis of this study [134] showed that 600-mg-clopidogrel loading dose compared with 300 mg had significantly lower 30-day unadjusted rates of definite or probable ST (1.7 % vs. 2.8 %, p = 0.04), as well as lower mortality (p = 0.03) and reinfarction (p = 0.02), and, without higher bleeding rates. Bivalirudin monotherapy resulted in similar reductions in net adverse cardiac event rates with both doses (p-interaction = 0.41). However, a 600-mg-clopidogrel loading dose was an independent predictor of lower rates of 30-day major adverse cardiac events (p = 0.04) [134].

In the setting of STEMI, current guidelines recommended bivalirudin over UFH and a GPI, restricting the use of GPI to bailout (Class I, LOE B) [49, 50]. In patients at high risk of bleeding the American guidelines recommended bivalirudin preferred over UFH with GPI (Class IIa, LOE B) [49] (Table 3.2).

Factor Xa Inhibitors

Fondaparinux

Mechanism of Action and Pharmacokinetic/Pharmacodynamic Profile

Fondaparinux is a selective indirect FXa inhibitor. This compound, with a molecular weight of 1,728 Da, is a synthetic analog of the unique AT-binding pentasaccharide sequence found in UFH. It binds reversibly to AT and provokes an irreversible conformational change at the reactive site of AT that increases its reactivity with FXa [135]. Fondaparinux is available to activate additional AT molecules after being released from AT, but it does not increase the rate of thrombin inhibition by AT because it is too short to bridge AT to thrombin. Fondaparinux does not have any inhibitory action against thrombin that is already formed, even though it inhibits FXa-dependent thrombin generation [113]. After SC injection the bioavailability is 100 % [136, 137]. The elimination half-life is 17 h with primary renal clearance. Fondaparinux is contraindicated in patients with severe renal impairment [40, 113, 138]. The anticoagulant response of fondaparinux is predictable and its PK profile is linear when it is given in SC doses of 2–8 mg or in IV doses ranging from 2 to 20 mg that result in anti-Xa activity that is roughly 7 times that of LMWHs [136, 137]. Its minimal nonspecific binding to plasma proteins it is likely to be the reason of its excellent bioavailability and predictable anticoagulant response [139].

Even if monitoring is not required, the anticoagulant effect of fondaparinux can be measured in anti-FXa units. Fondaparinux does not affect other parameters of anticoagulation, including aPTT, activated clotting time, or prothromb in time [138] and does not induce the formation of UFH:platelet factor-4 complexes and does not cross-react with HIT antibodies. Therefore, it is unlikely that induces HIT [140]. Not with Standing fondaparinux is not labeled for treatment of HIT, it has been used successfully to treat HIT patients [141, 142].It is unlikely that fondaparinux induces osteoporosis because it has no effect on osteoblasts [143]. In pregnancy, fondaparinux has not been studied enough, but it does not seem to cross the placental barrier [144].

Dosing, Monitoring, Reversal

Fondaparinux 2.5 mg daily was shown to have the best efficacy/safety profile when compared with 4-, 8-, and 12-mg doses of fondaparinux and with enoxaparin 1 mg/kg b.i.d based on a dose-ranging study of fondaparinux versus enoxaparin in the setting of UA/NSTEMI involving 1,147 patients [145].

There are no data about coagulation monitoring as part of the clinical development of this drug, but currently it is not recommended. Also in patients with severe renal impairment (CrCl <30 mL/min), fondaparinux has not been adequately studied. However, it is established that in patients with moderate renal impairment (30–50 mL/min) fondaparinux dose should be reduced in half or low-dose heparin should be used in place of fondaparinux [113]. To assess the anticoagulant effect of fondaparinux it is possible to measure anti-Xa levels, but the standard therapeutic level is unknown. It is important to highlight that protamine is not able to reverse the anticoagulant effect of fondaparinux. Recombinant factor VIIa may be given to achieve the reversal of the anticoagulant effect of fondaparinux if life-threatening bleeding takes place due to this agent [146].

Indications

Evidence for Use: UA/NSTEMI

The large-scale OASIS-5 trial (n = 20,078) evaluated the efficacy and safety of fondaparinux (2.5 mg SC daily) compared with enoxaparin (1 mg/kg SC b.i.d) in patients with UA/NSTEMI [147]. Fondaparinux demonstrated to be noninferior vs. enoxaparin in the primary outcome of combined death, MI, or refractory ischemia at 9 days was achieved (P = 0.007), with less incidence of major bleeding (P < 0.001). Fondaparinux showed a superior net clinical benefit (composite of death, MI refractory ischemia, or major bleeding) compared with enoxaparin (P < 0.001). Compared with enoxaparin, fondaparinux also demonstrated significantly a reduction in mortality at 6 months (P = 0.05). Nevertheless, more catheter-related thrombus formation occurred with fondaparinux in the group of patients who underwent PCI (P < 0.001), showing that anti-coagulation with fondaparinux alone is not enough for PCI, therefore another anticoagulant with FIIa activity (such as UFH) must be coadministered [147].

The main disadvantage of fondaparinux in this trial was the excess of catheter thrombosis seen in patients undergoing PCI (0.9 % vs. 0.4 % with enoxaparin), which has limited the widespread use of the drug in this setting. For that reason the OASIS investigators conducted The Fondaparinux Trial With UFH During Revascularization in ACS (FUTURA/OASIS-8) trial (n = 2,026) in order to evaluate the safety of 2 dose regimens of adjunctive IV UFH during PCI in high-risk patients with NSTEMI initially treated with fondaparinux [148]. Patients received either low-dose UFH (50 U/kg, regardless of use of GPI) or standard-dose UFH (85 U/kg or 60 U/kg with GPI), adjusted by activated clotting time. In terms of preventing peri-PCI major bleeding or major vascular access-site complications, low fixed-dose of UFH was not superior to standard ACT-guided UFH. Thrombotic events were not significantly different between the treatment groups (P = 0.27). Catheter thrombosis rates were very low (0.5 % in the low-dose group and 0.1 % in the standard-dose group, P = 0.15) [148].

Based on the above, current guidelines recommended 2.5 mg SC once daily as having the most favorable efficacy-safety profile with respect to anticoagulation (Class I, LOE A), avoiding its use for CrCl <30 mL/min. During PCI, at present2012 American guidelines recommend an additional 50–60 IU/kg IV bolus of UFH [40] while European guidelines recommend a 85 IU/kg IV bolus of UFH (adapted to ACT) or 60 IU in the case of concomitant use of GPI (Class I, LOE B) [41] (Table 3.1).

Evidence for Use: STEMI

In the OASIS-6 trial (n = 12,092), fondaparinux was evaluated as an alternative to standard adjunctive anticoagulation in patients with STEMI [149]. Patients received 2.5 mg SC daily for 8 day and it was compared with either no UFH (stratum I) or UFH infusion (stratum II) for 48 h. In approximately 25 % of patients primary PCI was performed. Approximately half the patients received fibrinolytic therapy, of whom 73 % received SK. In patients who received fondaparinux, the primary outcome of 30-day death or MI was significantly reduced (P = 0.008), although this was driven by patients in stratum I only. No significant benefit with fondaparinux was found in patients who underwent primary PCI or who were in stratum II. It is important to highlight that, compared with UFH, patients who underwent primary PCI with fondaparinux presented more catheter-related thrombi (P < 0.001), more coronary complications (P = 0.04), and a trend toward higher death or MI compared with UFH (P = 0.19).

Importantly, although European guidelines recommend using of fondaparinux in ACS [50], in the United States fondaparinux is not currently approved for such use by the FDA, as it is reflected in the current ACC guidelines for STEMI [49], because of the risk of catheter thrombosis (Class III, LOE: B) (Table 3.2).

As adjunctive antithrombotic therapy to support reperfusion with fibrinolytic therapy an initial IV dose of 2.5 mg of fondaparinux is recommended, and then 2.5 mg subcutaneously daily starting the following day for the index hospitalization up to 8 days or until revascularization. Fondaparinux is contraindicated if CrCl <30 mL/min [49] (Table 3.2).

Otamixaban

Otamixaban is a specific direct parenteral small molecule that inhibits clot-bound FXa which is inaccessible to large molecule or indirect inhibitors agent. Otamixaban is not still under advanced clinical investigation and not approved for clinical use. However, this agent has shown thus far promising results. Otamixaban has a very favorable PK/PD profile:

short acting (half-life30 min), weight based bolus (vs. infusion), no need for monitoring and no significant renal elimination (<25 %), but no antidote to otamixaban has been described [150].

In the Randomized, double-blind, dose-ranging study of otamixaban, a novel, parenteral, short-acting direct factor Xa inhibitor, in percutaneous coronary intervention (the SEPIA-PCI trial) [151], 947 patients were randomly assigned to either 1 of 5 weight-adjusted otamixaban regimens or weight-adjusted UFH before PCI. The study showed that otamixaban reduced the median change in prothrombin fragments $1+2$ (F1+2) significantly more than UFH at the highest dose regimen (P=0.008), without significant difference in the incidence of TIMI bleeding compared with UFH [151]. Posteriorly, another phase II study: the Otamixaban for the treatment of patients with non-ST-elevation acute coronary syndromes (SEPIA-ACS1 TIMI 42) trial (n=3,241) assessed the dose response on death, MI, urgent revascularization or bail-out in patients with NSTE-ACS with encouraging results about safety and efficacy, concluding that otamixaban 0.105–014 mg/kg/h appeared to be best range for further study as a replacement of UFH and GPI [152]. The ongoing phase III Treatment of Acute coronary syndromes with Otamixaban (TAO) trial (n=13,240) is evaluating the efficacy of otamixaban vs. UFH with and without eptifibatide on reduction of death or MI in patients with NSTE-ACS [153].

Oral Anticoagulant Therapy in ACS

The main reasons of the necessity of long term anticoagulation in ACS patients is the coexistence of another indication for anticoagulant therapy, such as atrial fibrillation (AF), left ventricular thrombus, advanced heart failure, deep venous thrombosis, prosthetic heart valves, or history of pulmonary embolism. The main risk in these patients remains the concomitant use of antiplatelet therapy and the consequent high risk of bleeding. Although, in the ACS population a considerable reduction in cardiovascular events is obtained with long-term dual antiplatelet therapy (DAPT) using aspirin and a $P2Y_{12}$ platelet receptor, [154] the risk of a recurrent vascular event within 12 months is still high and underscores the necessity of better secondary prevention strategies. Given that levels of thrombin generation persist elevated in ACS patients [155], and given the role of thrombin on arterial thrombogenesis, long-term use of oral anticoagulant strategies have been considered for secondary prevention of coronary events. Initially, vitamin K antagonists (VKAs) have been studied, mostly in combination with aspirin. However, despite the proven efficacy of this strategy, bleeding rates were high. The development of novel oral anticoagulants (NOACs) characterized by a better safety profile compared with VKAs have led to reconsider long-term oral anticoagulant therapy in adjunct to standard of care antiplatelet therapy, including mostly DAPT with aspirin and clopidogrel, also known as "triple therapy". The role of oral anticoagulant therapy for secondary prevention of ischemic events is described below.

Vitamin K Antagonists

VKAs, warfarin and coumarin derivatives, have demonstrated to reduce the risk of recurrent ischemic events both in monotherapy and in combination with aspirin [156]. In the Warfarin-Aspirin Re-Infarction Study (WARIS II) study, in combination with aspirin or given alone, warfarin was superior to aspirin alone in reducing the incidence of composite events after an acute MI but was associated with a higher risk of bleeding [156]. In this study, the combination therapy targeted an international normalized ratio (INR) of 2–2.5 and the warfarin alone group had a target INR of 2.8–4.2. No reduction in the combined risk of cardiovascular death, reinfarction, or stroke was demonstrated using a fixed, low dose of warfarin added to aspirin in the long term after MI, but this combination reduced the risk of stroke (secondary endpoint). An increased risk of bleeding was also associated to the concomitant administration of aspirin and warfarin [157].

These bleeding rates are even higher in patients who are on DAPT with aspirin and clopidogrel, as have been studied mostly in patients with AF undergoing PCI [158–160], the details of which going beyond the scope of this chapter which is focused on the role of anticoagulants for secondary prevention of ischemic recurrences in ACS.

Currently available data based on around 20,000 patients from randomized clinical trials show that oral anticoagulant therapy (given in adequate doses) reduce the rates of re-infarction and thromboembolic stroke, but increasing significantly the rates of hemorrhagic events [161]. Nevertheless, even in controlled trials the use of warfarin, presents several difficulties. For example, in the WARIS II study the INR was below target in about one third of patients, and those over 75 years of age were excluded [161].

Novel Oral Anticoagulants for Secondary Prevention

Several classes of NOACs have been developed. These agents have been primarily studied in patients with AF [162–164] and characterized by more favorable safety profile, particularly a lower risk of ICH, with comparable or better efficacy compared with VKAs. These agents also have the advantage of less drug-drug and food-drug interactions and that they can be administered in fixed doses without routine coagulation monitoring.

There are some aspects that should be considered for the periprocedural management of NOACs, compared with warfarin, such as their shorter half-life or the fact that the onset of their effects is within 2 h, provided that intestinal absorption is normal. Table 3.3 summarizes the recommendations for NOACs in patients undergoing elective PCI. The current status of knowledge of NOACs for secondary prevention of ischemic events in ACS is described below.

TABLE 3.3 Elective PCI recommendations

Renal function (CrCl mL/min)	Half life (hours)	Timing of Procedure after last dose of NOAC
Dabigatran		
>50 mL/min	15 (12–34)	24 h
>30 to ≤50 mL/min	18 (13–13)	2 days
≥30 mL/min	27 (22–35)	4 days
Rivaroxaban		
>30 mL/min	12 (11–13)	24 h
≤30 mL/min	Unknown	2 days
Apixaban		
>50 mL/min	7–8	24 h
<30 to ≤50 mL/min	17–18	2 days

Adapted from: Stangier et al. [165]; Schulman et al. [166]; Spyropoulos et al. [167]

Oral Direct Thrombin Inhibitors

Ximelagatran

The Efficacy and Safety of the Oral Direct Thrombin Inhibitor Ximelagatran in Patients with Recent Myocardial Damage (ESTEEM) trial for the secondary prevention of ACS showed a 24 % relative reduction with ximelagatran plus aspirin treatment for 6 months in the risk of the primary composite end point of death, nonfatal MI, and severe recurrent ischemia versus aspirin alone, although this occurred at the expense of an increased risk of bleeding [168]. Ximelagatran was retrieved from the market due to safety concerns (hepatic toxicity), but did provide encouraging results for other NOACs to be tested for secondary prevention in ACS.

Dabigatran Etexilate

Dabigatran etexilate binds reversibly and directly to the catalytic site of thrombin. It is a synthetic low molecular weight eptidomimetic generated as a prodrug which immediately after absorption is biotranformed by an esterase-mediated hydrolysis to the active compound dabigatran [169–171] Table 3.4 summarizes the principal pharmacologic characteristics of dabigatran etexilate compared with the new FXa inhibitors [173].

The Dose Finding Study for Dabigatran Etexilate in Patients With Acute Coronary Syndrome (RE-DEEM) trial (n = 1,861) was a phase II study that showed a dose-dependent increase in clinically relevant bleeding events, with highest rates with dose regimens currently used in AF (110 mg and 150 mg b.i.d.) [174]. Despite higher dabigatran doses compared with lower doses and placebo group seemed to have some benefit, it was impossible to demonstrate an efficacy difference in cardiovascular death, nonfatal MI or nonhemorrhagic stroke because the lack of enough statistical power of the trial [174]. Phase III clinical testing of dabigatran in ACS has not been pursued.

Oral Direct Factor Xa Inhibitors

Rivaroxaban, apixaban and darexaban are the three oral direct FXa inhibitors that have been most studied over recent years. Table 3.4 summarize the principal pharmacologic characteristics and dosages of these drugs compared with dabigatran [173, 175].

Darexaban (YM150)

The safety, tolerability, and regimen of darexaban for the prevention of ischemic events in ACS were evaluated in The Study Evaluating Safety, Tolerability and Efficacy of YM150 in Subjects With Acute Coronary Syndromes (RUBY-1) trial [176]. The study did not find benefits regarding an addition of

TABLE 3.4 Pharmacological characteristics of oral direct thrombin inhibitors and oral direct factor Xa inhibitors

	Dabigatran etexilate	Rivaroxaban	Apixaban	Darexaban
Mechanism of action	Selective direct thrombin (FIIa) inhibitor	Selective direct FXa inhibitor	Selective direct FXa inhibitor	Selective direct FXa inhibitor
Prodrug	Yes	No	No	Yes
Oral bioavailability	6.5 %	80–100 %	50–66 %	5 %
Half-life (hours)	12–17	5–13	8–15	14–18
Excretion	Renal 80 % Fecal 20 %	Renal 66 % 36 % unchanged 30 % inactive metabolites Fecal-biliary 28 %	Renal 27 % Fecal 55 %	Renal 50 % Fecal 50 %
Time to maximum inhibition (hours)	0.5–2	1–4	1–4	1–1.5
Potential metabolic drug interactions	P-glycoprotein Inhibitors of P-gp: Verapamil, reduce dose Dronedarone: avoid Potent inducers of P-gp[c]: avoid	CYP3A4/ P-glycoprotein Potent inhibitors of CYP3A4 and P-gp[a]: avoid Potent inducers of CYP3A4[b]and P-gp: use with caution	CYP3A4/P-glycoprotein Potent inhibitors of CYP3A4 and P-gp[a]: avoid Potent inducers of CYP3A4[b] and P-gp[c] use with caution	No drug-drug interactions with CYP3A4/ P-glycoprotein inhibitors and inducers

(continued)

TABLE 3.4 (continued)

	Dabigatran etexilate	Rivaroxaban	Apixaban	Darexaban
Reverse effect	Antidote not available Hemodialysis may remove 60 % Oral activated charcoal may adsorb it from the stomach. Inactivated or activated prothrombin complex concentrates or recombinant activated FVII may be useful if uncontrolled bleeding	Antidote not available Hemodialysis not effective (high plasma protein binding) Fresh frozen plasma, prothrombin complex concentrates, or activated FVII may reverse their effects		Antidote not available

Adapted from De Caterina et al. [172]

CYP cytochrome P450 isoenzyme, *F* factor, *P-gp* P-glycoprotein

[a]Potent inhibitors of CYP3A4 include antifungals (e.g. ketoconazole, intraconazole, voriconazole, posaconazole), chloramphenicol, clarithromycin, and protease inhibitors (e.g. ritonavir, atanazavir). P-gp inhibitors include verapamil, amiodarone, quinidine, and clarithromycin

[b]Potent CYP3A4 inducers include phenytoin, carbamazepine, phenobarbital, and St. John's wort

[c]P-gp inducers include rifampicin, St. John's wort (Hypericum perforatum), carbamazepine, and phenytoin

efficacy to DAPT in this setting, but showed an expected dose-related 2- to 4-fold increase in bleeding versus placebo as the only safety concern [176]. Darexaban development has been discontinued.

Apixaban

The phase II Apixaban for Prevention of Acute Ischemic and Safety Events (APPRAISE) trial found a dose-dependent interaction increased risk of bleeding complications with apixaban 2.5 mg b.i.d. and 10 mg q.d. Although apixaban was associated with a numerically lower incidence of cardiovascular death, MI, severe recurrent ischemia, or ischemic stroke it was not statistically significant [177]. APPRAISE-2 trial (n = 7,392) failed also to find similar benefits of adding a high dose of apixaban (5 mg b.i.d) to single or DAPT in a very-high-risk ACS population [178]. A greater number of intracranial and fatal bleeding events happened with apixaban than with placebo, without a significant reduction in recurrent ischemic events. Because of the wide CIs allow for either benefit or harm, the overall efficacy/safety balance of apixaban is still unknown.

Rivaroxaban

The Rivaroxaban in Combination With Aspirin Alone or With Aspirin and a thienopyridine in Patients With Acute Coronary Syndromes-TIMI 46 (ATLAS ACS-TIMI 46) trial [179], demonstrated either in patients receiving aspirin alone and in patients receiving DAPT, a rivaroxaban dose-dependent increased risk of clinically significant bleeding complications. However, the lower doses were associated with lowest bleeding risk and accompanied by an ischemic benefit. This set the basis for developing the phase III ATLAS ACS-2–TIMI 51 (ATLAS-2) trial (n = 15,526) demonstrated that both rivaroxaban regimens (2.5-mg and 5-mg b.i.d.) compared with placebo significantly reduced the primary efficacy composite of cardiovascular death, MI, or stroke (p < 0.008) [180, 181]. The 2.5-mg (but not 5-mg b.i.d.), reduced cardiovascular and all-cause mortality. The 5 mg b.i.d. (but not 2.5-mg b.i.d.) reduced MI. Both dosages of rivaroxaban reduced significantly the risk of ST, as compared with placebo ($P = 0.02$), while the 2.5-mg b.i.d dose showed a nonsignificant but directionally consistent benefit for MI. The rates of non-CABG-related TIMI major bleeding and ICH with both doses were significantly increased, without a significant increase in fatal bleeding ($P = 0.66$) [180, 181].

Current ESC Guidelines for the management of STEMI recommended considering the use of low-dose rivaroxaban (2.5 mg b.i.d) in selected patients who receive aspirin and clopidogrel, if the patient is at low bleeding risk (Class of recommendation IIb, LOE B) [50]. Rivaroxaban however is still not approved for clinical use in the United States.

Anticoagulants Under Clinical Development

Aptamers are small oligonucleotides that form unique sequence-dependent three-dimensional structures [182, 183] and can be developed to inhibit specific protein targets with high affinity and used as active drugs. Aptamers provide the code for their own complement (reversal agent), which can be developed and used to inhibit their function [183–185]. Reversal of aptamer activity can be titrated to the patient's clinical condition given that the degree of reversal is directly related to the molar ratio of administered components. The REG1 anticoagulation system is a novel, aptamer-based, FIXa inhibitor that is being described for use in patients undergoing PCI. This system consists of pegnivacogin, a single-stranded RNA factor IXa inhibitor, and its complementary reversal agent, anivamersen, which binds to and inactivates pegnivacogin with rapid kinetics [186]. Phase I [185–188] and phase II [189] studies investigated REG1 with encouraging results. Recently, the RADAR (A Randomized, Partially Blinded, Multicenter, Active-Controlled, Dose-Ranging Study Assessing the Safety, Efficacy, and Pharmacodynamics of the REG1 Anticoagulation System in

Patients with ACS) trial [190, 191] showed that at least 50 % anivamersen-mediated reversal of pegnivacogin was necessary to effectively diminish bleeding after early femoral sheath removal in invasively managed patients with ACS. To determine the safety and efficacy of REG1 more powered randomized clinical trials are needed. A large scale phase III clinical trial is currently planned.

Thrombin generation is also decreased by drugs that target coagulation proteases that drive the propagation phase. Coagulation proteases modulate inflammation by activating protease activated receptors (PARs), and by binding to other cell surface receptors, such as Thrombomodulin (TM) and endothelial protein C receptor (EPCR) [192, 193]. PAR-2 does not bind thrombin, but the tissue factor (TF)/FVIIa complex and FXa can activate this receptor [194]. Activation of PARs by the various coagulation proteases results in the upregulation of genes involved in inflammation, including interleukin (IL)-8 and tumour necrosis factor (TNF)-α. TF/FVIIa-induced signaling events can modulate cell fate and behaviour, rendering cells and tissues proliferative, promigratory, and resistant to apoptosis. Based on these findings, PAR inhibitors are under development and PAR-1-targeting drugs have undergone phase III clinical trial evaluation [195, 196]. In addition to the role of PARs in inflammation, additional cross-talk occurs at the level of FXa. This concept is highlighted by the recent demonstration that lufaxin, a FXa inhibitor from the salivary glands of blood-sucking arthropods, not only inhibits thrombosis in mice, but also attenuates oedema formation triggered by FXa injection into their paws [197]. Other anticoagulant therapies in development that block target coagulationproteases that drive the propagation phase, such as FVIIIa (TB-402), or jointly FVa/FVIIIa, cofactors that are critical for the generation of thrombin (drotrecogin, which is a recombinant form of human activated protein C and recomodulin and solulin, both of which are recombinant soluble derivatives of human thrombomodulin). Inhibitors toward the TF/FVIIa complex, such as recombinant TFPI (tifacogin), recombinant nematode anticoagulant

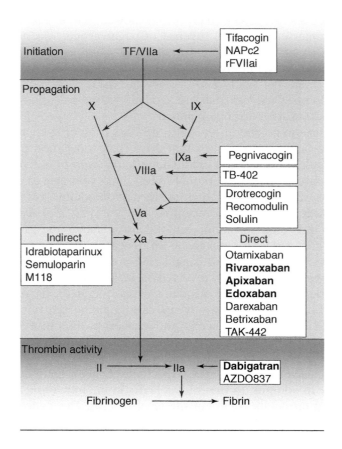

protein (NAP)C2, active site–inhibited recombinant (r) FVIIa inhibitors (rFVIIaI) and monoclonal antibodies against TFT have been developed to target the initiation of coagulation [107] (Fig. 3.4).

Conclusions

During the last decade antithrombotic treatment of ACS has changed very rapidly, particularly due to the development of new antiplatelet and anticoagulant agents. The coagulation

FIGURE 3.4 Targets of Novel Anticoagulants. Compared with the indirect thrombin inhibitors (such as the heparins), direct thrombin inhibitors (DTIs) bind directly to thrombin and prevent fibrin formation as well as thrombin-mediated activation of factor (F) V, FVIII, FXI, and FXIII. Hirudin, bivalirudin, and argatroban are the available parenteral DTIs. Oral DTIs including ximelagatran (withdrawn from development), AZD0837 (under evaluation), and dabigatran etexilate, are prodrugs that generate an active compound able to bind directly to the catalytic site of thrombin. Other agents block target coagulation proteases that drive the propagation phase: FIXa (DNA aptamer pegnivacogin), FVIIIa (TB-402), or jointly FVa/FVIIIa, cofactors for the generation of thrombin (drotrecogin, recomodulin and solulin). Inhibitors toward the tissue factor/FVIIa complex, such as recombinant TFPI (tifacogin), recombinant nematode anticoagulant protein (NAP)C2, active site–inhibited recombinant (r) FVIIa inhibitors (rFVIIaI) and monoclonal antibodies against TFT have been developed to target the initiation of coagulation (Reproduced from De Caterina et al. [172])

←_____

cascade offers numerous potential targets of treatment that allow interfering in many processes of haemostasis and thrombosis. Currently, there are a plethora of new parenteral and oral anticoagulants that are being developed and incorporated into clinical practice in the setting of ACS. Many of these are preferred over older treatment regimens because of their more favorable safety profile. However, others still require to be refined and ongoing clinical trials will provide more insights on the safety and efficacy of these strategies.

Acknowledgements   Ana Muñiz-Lozano is recipient of a training grant from the Spanish Society of Cardiology ("Beca de la Sección de Cardiopatía Isquémica para Formación e Investigación Post Residencia en el Extranjero" – Sociedad Española de Cardiología).

Disclosures

Dominick J. Angiolillo has received payment as an individual for: (a) Consulting fee or honorarium from Bristol Myers Squibb, Sanofi-Aventis, Eli Lilly, Daiichi Sankyo, The Medicines Company, AstraZeneca, Merck, Evolva, Abbott Vascular and PLx Pharma; (b) Participation in review activities from Johnson & Johnson, St. Jude, and Sunovion. Institutional payments for grants from Bristol Myers Squibb, Sanofi-Aventis, Glaxo Smith Kline, Otsuka, Eli Lilly, Daiichi Sankyo, The Medicines Company, AstraZeneca, Evolva; and has other financial relationships with Esther and King Biomedical Research Grant.

Ana Muñiz-Lozano: has no conflict of interest to report.

Fabiana Rollini: has no conflict of interest to report.

Francesco Franchi: has no conflict of interest to report.

References

1. Davies MJ, Thomas AC. Plaque fissuring-the cause of acute myocardial infarction, sudden ischaemic death, and crescendo angina. Br Heart J. 1985;53:363–73.
2. Farb A, Burke AP, Tang AL, et al. Coronary plaque erosion without rupture into a lipid core. A frequent cause of coronary thrombosis in sudden coronary death. Circulation. 1996;93(7):1354–63.
3. Braunwald E. Unstable angina and non-ST elevation myocardial infarction. Am J Respir Crit Care Med. 2012;185:924–32.
4. Furie B, Furie BC. Molecular and cellular biology of blood coagulation. N Engl J Med. 1992;326:800–6.
5. Chesebro JH, Zoldhelyi P, Badimon L, et al. Role of thrombin in arterial thrombosis: implications for therapy. Thromb Haemost. 1991;66:1–5.
6. Bar-Shavit R, Eldor A, Vlodavsky I. Binding of thrombin to subendothelial extracellular matrix: protection and expression of functional properties. J Clin Invest. 1989;84:1096–104.
7. Hogg PJ, Jackson CM. Fibrin monomer protects thrombin from inactivation by heparin-antithrombin III: implications for heparin efficacy. Proc Natl Acad Sci USA. 1989;86:3619–23.
8. Weitz JI, Hudoba M, Massel D, et al. Clot-bound thrombin is protected from inhibition by heparinantithrombin III but is susceptible to inactivation by antithrombin III-independent inhibitors. J Clin Invest. 1990;86:385–91.
9. Weitz JI, Leslie B, Hudoba M. Thrombin binds to soluble fibrin degradation products where it is protected from inhibition by heparin-antithrombin but susceptible to inactivation by antithrombin- independent inhibitors. Circulation. 1998;97:544–52.
10. Serruys P, Vranckx P, Allikmets K, et al. Clinical development of bivalirudin (angiox): rationale for thrombin-specific anticoagulation in percutaneous coronary intervention and acute coronary syndromes. Int J Clin Pract. 2006;60:344–50.

11. De Caterina R, Husted S, Wallentin L, et al. General mechanisms of coagulation and targets of anticoagulants (Section I). Position Paper of the ESC Working Group on Thrombosis – Task Force on Anticoagulants in Heart Disease. Thromb Haemost. 2013;109:569–79.
12. Di Nisio M, Middeldorp S, Buller HR. Direct thrombin inhibitors. N Engl J Med. 2005;353:1028–40.
13. McAllister BM, Demis DJ. Heparin metabolism: isolation and characterization of uroheparin. Nature. 1966;212:293–4.
14. Hirsh J. Heparin. N Engl J Med. 1992;324:1565–74.
15. Hull RD, Raskob GE, Hirsh J, et al. Continuous intravenous heparin compared with intermittent SC heparin in the initial treatment of proximal-vein thrombosis. N Engl J Med. 1986;315:1109–14.
16. Hirsh J, van Aken WG, Gallus AS, et al. Heparin kinetics in venous thrombosis and pulmonary embolism. Circulation. 1976;53:691–5.
17. Young E, Prins M, Levine MN, et al. Heparin binding to plasma proteins, an important mechanism for heparin resistance. Thromb Haemost. 1992;67:639–43.
18. Barzu T, Molho P, Tobelem G, et al. Binding and endocytosis of heparin by human endothelial cells in culture. Biochim Biophys Acta. 1985;845:196–203.
19. Sobel M, McNeill PM, Carlson PL, et al. Heparin inhibition of von Willebrand factordependent platelet function in vitro and in vivo. J Clin Invest. 1991;87:1787–93.
20. Friedman Y, Arsenis C. Studies on the heparin sulphamidase activity from rat spleen. Intracellular distribution and characterization of the enzyme. Biochem J. 1974;139:699–708.
21. Dawes J, Papper DS. Catabolism of low-dose heparin in man. Thromb Res. 1979;14:845–60.
22. de Swart CA, Nijmeyer B, Roelofs JM, et al. Kinetics of intravenously administered heparin in normal humans. Blood. 1982;60:1251–8.
23. Olsson P, Lagergren H, Ek S. The elimination from plasma of intravenous heparin. An experimental study on dogs and humans. Acta Med Scand. 1963;173:619–30.
24. Bjornsson TD, Wolfram KM, Kitchell BB. Heparin kinetics determined by three assay methods. Clin Pharmacol Ther. 1982;31:104–13.
25. Theroux P, Ouimet H, McCans J, et al. Aspirin, heparin, or both to treat acute unstable angina. N Engl J Med. 1988;319:1105–11.
26. Granger CB, Miller JM, Bovill EG, et al. Rebound increase in thrombin generation and activity after cessation of intravenous heparin in patients with acute coronary syndromes. Circulation. 1995;91:1929–35.
27. Theroux P, Waters D, Lam J, et al. Reactivation of unstable angina after the discontinuation of heparin. N Engl J Med. 1992;327:141–5.
28. Heiden D, Mielke Jr CH, Rodvien R. Impairment by heparin of primary haemostasis and platelet [14C]5-hydroxytryptamine release. Br J Haematol. 1977;36:427–36.

29. Eika C. Inhibition of thrombin-induced aggregation of human platelets by heparin and antithrombin 3. Scand J Haematol. 1971;8:250–6.

30. Kelton JG, Hirsh J. Bleeding associated with antithrombotic therapy. Semin Hematol. 1980;17:259–91.

31. Blajchman MA, Young E, Ofosu FA. Effects of unfractionated heparin, dermatan sulfate and low molecular weight heparin on vessel wall permeability in rabbits. Ann N Y Acad Sci. 1989;556:245–54.

32. Clowes AW, Karnowsky MJ. Suppression by heparin of smooth muscle cell proliferation in injured arteries. Nature. 1977;265:625–6.

33. Castellot Jr JJ, Favreau LV, Karnovsky MJ, et al. Inhibition of vascular smooth muscle cell growth by endothelial cell-derived heparin. Possible role of a platelet endoglycosidase. J Biol Chem. 1982;257:11256–60.

34. Shaughnessy SG, Young E, Deschamps P, et al. The effects of low molecular weight and standard heparin on calcium loss from fetal rat calvaria. Blood. 1995;86:1368–73.

35. Bhandari M, Hirsh J, Weitz JI, et al. The effects of standard and low molecular weight heparin on bone nodule formation in vitro. Thromb Haemost. 1998;80:413–7.

36. Visentin GP, Ford SE, Scott JP, et al. Antibodies from patients with heparin-induced thrombocytopenia/thrombosis are specific for platelet factor 4 complexed with heparin or bound to endothelial cells. J Clin Invest. 1994;93:81–8.

37. Greinacher A, Liebenhoff U, Kiefel V, et al. Heparin-associated thrombocytopenia: the effects of various intravenous IgG preparations on antibody mediated platelet activation -a possible new indication for high dose i.v. IgG. Thromb Haemost. 1994;71:641–5.

38. Whitfield LR, Lele AS, Levy G. Effect of pregnancy on the relationship between concentration and anticoagulant action of heparin. Clin Pharmacol Ther. 1983;34:23–8.

39. Edson JR, Krivit W, White JG. Kaolin partial thromboplastin time: high levels of procoagulants producing short clotting times or masking deficiencies of other procoagulants or low concentrations of anticoagulants. J Lab Clin Med. 1967;70:463–70.

40. Jneid H, Anderson JL, Wright RS, et al. 2012 ACCF/AHA focused update of the guideline for the management of patients with unstable angina/Non-ST-elevation myocardial infarction (updating the 2007 guideline and replacing the 2011 focused update): a report of the American College of Cardiology Foundation/American Heart Association Task Force on practice guidelines. Circulation. 2012;126:875–910.

41. Hamm CW, Bassand JP, Agewall S, et al. 2011 ESC Guidelines for the management of acute coronary syndromes in patients presenting without persistent ST-segment elevation: The Task Force for the management of acute coronary syndromes (ACS) in patients

presenting without persistent ST-segment elevation of the European Society of Cardiology (ESC). Eur Heart. 2011;J32:2999–3054.

42. Telford AM, Wilson C. Trial of heparin versus atenolol in prevention of myocardial infarction in intermediate coronary syndrome. Lancet. 1981;1:1225–8.

43. Williams DO, Kirby MG, McPherson K, et al. Anticoagulant treatment of unstable angina. Br J Clin Pract. 1986;40:114–6.

44. Theroux P, Waters D, Qiu S, et al. Aspirin versus heparin to prevent myocardial infarction during the acute phase of unstable angina. Circulation. 1993;88:2045–8.

45. Neri Serneri GG, Gensini GF, Poggesi L, et al. Effect of heparin, aspirin, or alteplase in reduction of myocardial ischaemia in refractory unstable angina. Lancet. 1990;335:615–8.

46. Holdright D, Patel D, Cunningham D, et al. Comparison of the effect of heparin and aspirin versus aspirin alone on transient myocardial ischemia and in-hospital prognosis in patients with unstable angina. J Am Coll Cardiol. 1994;24:39–45.

47. Cohen M, Adams PC, Hawkins L, et al. Usefulness of antithrombotic therapy in resting angina pectoris or non-Q-wave myocardial infarction in preventing death and myocardial infarction (a pilot study from the Antithrombotic Therapy in Acute Coronary Syndromes Study Group). Am J Cardiol. 1990;66:1287–92.

48. Oler A, Whooley MA, Oler J, et al. Adding heparin to aspirin reduces the incidence of myocardial infarction and death in patients with unstable angina. A meta-analysis. JAMA. 1996;276:811–5.

49. O'Gara PT, Kushner FG, Ascheim DD, et al. 2013 ACCF/AHA guideline for the management of ST-elevation myocardial infarction: a report of the American College of Cardiology Foundation/ American Heart Association Task Force on Practice Guidelines. Circulation. 2013;127:e362–425.

50. Steg PG, James SK, Atar D, Badano LP, et al. ESC Guidelines for the management of acute myocardial infarction in patients presenting with ST-segment elevation. Task Force on the management of ST-segment elevation acute myocardial infarction of the European Society of Cardiology (ESC). Eur Heart J. 2012;33:2569–619.

51. Antman EM, Morrow DA, McCabe CH, et al. Enoxaparin versus unfractionated heparin with fibrinolysis for ST-elevation myocardial infarction. N Engl J Med. 2006;354:1477–88.

52. Hirsh J, Warkentin TE, Raschke R, et al. Heparin and low-molecular-weight heparin: mechanisms of action, pharmacokinetics, dosing considerations, monitoring, efficacy, and safety. Chest. 1998;114:489S–510.

53. Hochman JS, Wali AU, Gavrila D, et al. A new regimen for heparin use in acute coronary syndromes. Am Heart J. 1999;138:313–8.

54. Morabia A. Heparin doses and major bleedings. Lancet. 1986;1:1278–9.

55. Antman EM. Hirudin in acute myocardial infarction. Safety report from the Thrombolysis and Thrombin Inhibition in Myocardial Infarction (TIMI) 9A Trial. Circulation. 1994;90:1624–30.
56. Warkentin TE, Levine MN, Hirsh J, et al. Heparin-induced thrombo-cytopenia in patients treated with low-molecular-weight heparin or unfractionated heparin. N Engl J Med. 1995;332:1330–5.
57. Antman EM. Hirudin in acute myocardial infarction. Thrombolysis and Thrombin Inhibition in Myocardial Infarction (TIMI) 9B trial. Circulation. 1996;94:911–21.
58. The Global Use of Strategies to Open Occluded Coronary Arteries (GUSTO) IIa Investigators. Randomized trial of intravenous hepa-rin versus recombinant hirudin for acute coronary syndromes. Circulation. 1994;90:1631–7.
59. The Global Use of Strategies to Open Occluded Coronary Arteries (GUSTO) IIb Investigators. A comparison of recombinant hirudin with heparin for the treatment of acute coronary syndromes. N Engl J Med. 1996;335:775–82.
60. The EPIC Investigators. Use of a monoclonal antibody directed against the platelet glycoprotein IIb/IIIa receptor in high-risk coro-nary angioplasty. N Engl J Med. 1994;330:956–61.
61. Arepally GM, Ortel TL. Clinical practice. Heparin-induced throm-bocytopenia. N Engl J Med. 2006;355:809–17.
62. Baroletti SA, Goldhaber SZ. Heparin-induced thrombocytopenia. Circulation. 2006;114:e355–6.
63. Caplan SN, Berkman EM. Protamine sulfate and fish allergy. N Engl J Med. 1976;295:172.
64. Stewart WJ, McSweeney SM, Kellett MA, et al. Increased risk of severe protamine reactions in NPH insulin-dependent diabetics undergoing cardiac catheterization. Circulation. 1984;70:788–92.
65. Levine GN, Bates ER, Blankenship JC, et al. 2011 ACCF/AHA/SCAI guideline for percutaneous coronary intervention. A report of the American College of Cardiology Foundation/American Heart Association Task Force on Practice Guidelines and the Society for Cardiovascular Angiography and Interventions. J Am Coll Cardiol. 2011;58:e44–122.
66. Hirsh J, Anand SS, Halperin JL, et al. Mechanism of action and phar-macology of unfractionated heparin. Arterioscler Thromb Vasc Biol. 2001;21:1094–6.
67. Handeland GF, Abildgaard U, Holm HA, et al. Dose adjusted hepa-rin treatment of deep venous thrombosis: a comparison of unfrac-tionated and low molecular weight heparin. Eur J Clin Pharmacol. 1990;39:107–12.
68. Hirsh J, Levine MN. Low molecular weight heparin. Blood. 1992;79:1–17.
69. Weitz JI. Low-molecular-weight heparins. N Engl J Med. 1997;337:688–98.
70. Boneu B, Caranobe C, Cadroy Y, et al. Pharmacokinetic studies of standard unfractionated heparin, and low molecular weight heparins in the rabbit. Semin Thromb Hemost. 1988;14:18–27.

71. Brophy DF, Wazny LD, Gehr TW, et al. The pharmacokinetics of subcutaneous enoxaparin in end-stage renal disease. Pharmacotherapy. 2001;21:169–74.

72. Becker RC, Spencer FA, Gibson M, et al. Influence of patient characteristics and renal function on factor Xa inhibition pharmacokinetics and pharmacodynamics after enoxaparin administration in non-ST-segment elevation acute coronary syndromes. Am Heart J. 2002;143:753–9.

73. Samama MM, Poller L. Contemporary laboratory monitoring of low molecular weight heparins. Clin Lab Med. 1995;15:119–23.

74. Boneu B, de Moerloose P. How and when to monitor a patient treated with ow molecular weight heparin. Semin Thromb Hemost. 2001;27:519–22.

75. Johnson EA, Kirkwood TB, Stirling Y, et al. Brozovic M. Four heparin preparations: anti Xa potentiating effect of heparin after subcutaneous injection. Thromb Haemost. 1976;35:586–91.

76. Choay J, Petitou M, Lormeau JC, et al. Structure-activity relationship in heparin: a synthetic pentasaccharide with high affinity for antithrombin III and eliciting high anti-factor Xa activity. Biochem Biophys Res Commun. 1983;116:492–9.

77. Bara I., Samama M. Pharmacokinetics of low molecular weight heparins. Acta Chir Scand Suppl. 1988;543:65–72.

78. Bradbrook ID, Magnani HN, Moelker HC, et al. ORG 10172: a low molecular weight heparinoid anticoagulant with a long half-life in man. Br J Clin Pharmacol. 1987;23:667–75.

79. Antman EM, Cohen M, Radley D, et al. Assessment of the treatment effect of enoxaparin for unstable angina/non-Q-wave myocardial infarction. TIMI 11B-ESSENCE meta-analysis. Circulation. 1999;100:1602–8.

80. The Thrombolysis in Myocardial Infarction (TIMI) 11A Trial Investigators. Dose-ranging trial of enoxaparin for unstable angina: results of TIMI 11A. J Am Coll Cardiol. 1997;29:1474–82.

81. Bruno R, Baille P, Retout S, et al. Population pharmacokinetics and pharmacodynamics of enoxaparin in unstable angina and non-ST-segment elevation myocardial infarction. Br J Clin Pharmacol. 2003;56:407–14.

82. Warkentin TE, Roberts RS, Hirsh J, et al. An improved definition of immune heparininduced thrombocytopenia in postoperative orthopedic patients. Arch Intern Med. 2003;163:2518–24.

83. Greinacher A, Michels I, Mueller-Eckhardt C. Heparin-associated thrombocytopenia: the antibody is not heparin specific. Thromb Haemost. 1992;67:545–9.

84. Monreal M, Vinas L, Monreal L, et al. Heparin-related osteoporosis in rats. A comparative study between unfractionated heparin and a low-molecular-weight heparin. Haemostasis. 1990;20:204–7.

85. Racanelli A, Fareed J, Walenga JM, et al. Biochemical and pharmacologic studies on the protamine interactions with heparin, its fractions and fragments. Semin Thromb Hemost. 1985;11:176–89.

86. Wong GC, Giugliano RP, Antman EM. Use of low-molecular-weight heparins in the management of acute coronary artery syndromes and percutaneous coronary intervention. JAMA. 2003;289:331–42.
87. Klein W, Buchwald A, Hillis SE, et al. Comparison of low-molecular-weight heparin with unfractionated heparin acutely and with placebo for 6 weeks in the management of unstable coronary artery disease. Fragmin in unstable coronary artery disease study (FRIC). Circulation. 1997;96:61–8.
88. Fragmin During Instability in Coronary Artery Disease (FRISC) Study Group. Low-molecular-weight heparin during instability in coronary artery disease. Lancet. 1996;347:561–8.
89. FRAX.I.S. (FRAxiparine in Ischaemic Syndrome) Investigators. Comparison of two treatment durations (6 days and 14 days) of a low molecular weight heparin with a 6-day treatment of unfractionated heparin in the initial management of unstable angina or non-Q wave myocardial infarction. Eur Heart J. 1999;20:1553–62.
90. Ferguson JJ, Califf RM, Antman EM, et al. Enoxaparin vs. unfractionated heparin in high-risk patients with non-ST-segment elevation acute coronary syndromes managed with an intended early invasive strategy: primary results of the SYNERGY randomized trial. JAMA. 2004;292:45–54.
91. Cohen M, Demers C, Gurfinkel E, et al. A comparison of low-molecular-weight heparin with unfractionated heparin for unstable coronary artery disease. N Engl J Med. 1997;337:447–52.
92. Antman EM, McCabe CH, Gurfinkel EP, et al. Enoxaparin prevents death and cardiac ischemic events in unstable angina/non-Q-wave myocardial infarction. Results of the thrombolysis in myocardial infarction (TIMI) 11B trial. Circulation. 1999;100:1593–601.
93. Cohen M, Theroux P, Borzak S, et al. Randomized double-blind safety study of enoxaparin versus unfractionated heparin in patients with non-ST-segment elevation acute coronary syndromes treated with tirofiban and aspirin: the ACUTE II study. The Antithrombotic Combination Using Tirofiban and Enoxaparin. Am Heart J. 2002;144:470–7.
94. Goodman SG, Fitchett D, Armstrong PW, et al. Randomized evaluation of the safety and efficacy of enoxaparin versus unfractionated heparin in high-risk patients with non-ST-segment elevation acute coronary syndromes receiving the glycoprotein IIb/IIIa inhibitor eptifibatide. Circulation. 2003;107:238–44.
95. Blazing MA, de Lemos JA, White HD, et al. Safety and efficacy of enoxaparin vs. unfractionated heparin in patients with non-ST-segment elevation acute coronary syndromes who receive tirofiban and aspirin: a randomized controlled trial. JAMA. 2004;292:55–64.
96. Antman EM. The search for replacements for unfractionated heparin. Circulation. 2001;103:2310–4.

97. Petersen JL, Mahaffey KW, Hasselblad V, et al. Efficacy and bleeding complications among patients randomized to enoxaparin or unfractionated heparin for antithrombins therapy in non-ST-Segment elevation acute coronary syndromes: a systematic overview. JAMA. 2004;292:89–96.
98. The ASSENT-3 Investigators. Efficacy and safety of tenecteplase in combination with enoxaparin, abciximab, or unfractionated heparin: the ASSENT-3 randomised trial in acute myocardial infarction. Lancet. 2001;358:605–13.
99. Wallentin L, Goldstein P, Armstrong PW, et al. Efficacy and safety of tenecteplase in combination with the low-molecular-weight heparin enoxaparin or unfractionated heparin in the prehospital setting: the Assessment of the Safety and Efficacy of a New Thrombolytic Regimen (ASSENT)-3 PLUS randomized trial in acute myocardial infarction. Circulation. 2003;108:135–42.
100. Giraldez RR, Nicolau JC, Corbalan R, et al. Enoxaparin is superior to unfractionated heparin in patients with ST elevation myocardial infarction undergoing fibrinolysis regardless of the choice of lytic: an ExTRACT-TIMI 25 analysis. Eur Heart J. 2007;28:1566–73.
101. White HD, Braunwald E, Murphy SA, et al. Enoxaparin vs. unfractionated heparin with fibrinolysis for ST-elevation myocardial infarction in elderly and younger patients: results from ExTRACT-TIMI 25. Eur Heart J. 2007;28:1066–71.
102. Montalescot G, White HD, Gallo R, et al. STEEPLE Investigators. Enoxaparin versus unfractionated heparin in elective percutaneous coronary intervention. N Engl J Med. 2006;355:1058–60.
103. Antman EM, Louwerenburg HW, Baars HF, et al. Enoxaparin as adjunctive antithrombin therapy for ST-elevation myocardial infarction: results of the ENTIRE-Thrombolysis in Myocardial Infarction (TIMI) 23 Trial. Circulation 105:1642–9. Erratum in. Circulation. 2002;105:2799.
104. Gibson CM, Murphy SA, Montalescot G, et al. Percutaneous coronary intervention in patients receiving enoxaparin or unfractionated heparin after fibrinolytic therapy for ST-segment elevation myocardial infarction in the ExTRACT-TIMI 25 trial. J Am Coll Cardiol. 2007;49:2238–46.
105. Levine MN, Raskob G, Beyth RJ, et al. Hemorrhagic complications of anticoagulant treatment: The Seventh ACCP Conference on Antithrombotic and Thrombolytic Therapy. Chest. 2004;126:287S–310.
106. Eisert WG, Hauel N, Stangier J, et al. Dabigatran: an oral novel potent reversible nonpeptide inhibitor of thrombin. Arterioscler Thromb Vasc Biol. 2010;30:1885–9.
107. Weitz JI. Factor Xa and thrombin as targets for new oral anticoagulants. Thromb Res. 2011;127:S5–12.
108. Bates SM, Weitz JI. Direct thrombin inhibitors for treatment of arterial thrombosis: potential differences between bivalirudin and hirudin. Am J Cardiol. 1998;82:12P–8.

109. Xiao Z, Theroux P. Platelet activation with unfractionated heparin at therapeutic concentrations and comparisons with a low-molecular-weight heparin and with a direct thrombin inhibitor. Circulation. 1998;97:251–6.

110. Sorensen B, Ingerslev J. A direct thrombin inhibitor studied by dynamic whole blood clot formation. Haemostatic response to ex-vivo addition of recombinant factor VIIa or activated prothrombin complex concentrate. Thromb Haemost. 2006;96:446–53.

111. Wallis RB. Hirudins: from leeches to man. Semin Thromb Hemost. 1996;22:185–96.

112. OASIS-2 Investigators. Effects of recombinant hirudin (lepirudin) compared with heparin on death, myocardial infarction, refractory angina, and revascularisation procedures in patients with acute myocardial ischaemia without ST elevation: A randomised trial. Lancet. 1999;353:429–38.

113. Garcia DA, Baglin TP, Weitz JI, et al. Parenteral anticoagulants: Antithrombotic Therapy and Prevention of Thrombosis, 9th ed: American College of Chest Physicians Evidence-Based Clinical Practice Guidelines. Chest. 2012;141:e24S–43.

114. Lefevre G, Duval M, Gauron S, et al. Effect of renal impairment on the pharmacokinetics and pharmacodynamics of desirudin. Clin Pharmacol Ther. 1997;62:50–9.

115. Banner DW, Hadvary P. Inhibitor binding to thrombin: x-ray crystallographic studies. Adv Exp Med Biol. 1993;340:27–33.

116. Hursting MJ, Alford KL, Becker JC, et al. Novastan (brand of argatroban): a small molecule, direct thrombin inhibitor. Semin Thromb Hemost. 1997;23:503–16.

117. Lewis BE, Wallis DE, Leya F, et al. Argatroban-915 Investigators. Argatroban anticoagulation in patients with heparin-induced thrombocytopenia. Arch Intern Med. 2003;163:1849–56.

118. Swan SK, Hursting MJ. The pharmacokinetics and pharmacodynamics of argatroban: effects of age, gender, and hepatic or renal dysfunction. Pharmacotherapy. 2000;20:318–29.

119. Maraganore JM, Bourdon P, Jablonski J, et al. Design and characterization of hirulogs: a novel class of bivalent peptide inhibitors of thrombin. Biochemistry. 1990;29:7095–101.

120. Skrzypczak-Jankun E, Carperos VE, Ravichandran KG, et al. Structure of the hirugen and hirulog 1 complexes of alpha-thrombin. J Mol Biol. 1991;221:1379–93.

121. Witting JI, Bourdon P, Brezniak DV, et al. Thrombinspecific inhibition by and slow cleavage of hirulog-1. Biochem J. 1992;283:737–43.

122. Fox I, Dawson A, Loynds P, et al. Anticoagulant activity of Hirulog, a direct thrombin inhibitor, in humans. Thromb Haemost. 1993;69:157–63.

123. Robson R, White H, Aylward P, et al. Bivalirudin pharmacokinetics and pharmacodynamics: effect of renal function, dose, and gender. Clin Pharmacol Ther. 2002;71:433–9.

124. Chew DP, Bhatt DL, Kimball W, et al. Bivalirudin provides increasing benefit with decreasing renal function: a meta-analysis of randomized trials. Am J Cardiol. 2003;92:919–23.
125. Stone G, McLaurin BT, Cox DA, et al. ACUITY Investigators. Bivalirudin for patients with acute coronary syndromes. N Engl J Med. 2006;355:2203–16.
126. Kastrati A, Neumann FJ, Schulz S, et al. Abciximab and heparin versus bivalirudin for non-ST-elevation myocardial infarction. ISAR REACT 4 trial. New Engl J Med. 2011;365:1980–9.
127. Stone GW, Witzenbichler B, Guagliumi G, et al. Bivalirudin during primary PCI in acute myocardial infarction. N Engl J Med. 2008;358:2218–30.
128. Wasowicz M, Vegas A, Borger MA, et al. Bivalirudin anticoagulation for cardiopulmonary bypass in a patient with heparin-induced thrombocytopenia. Can J Anaesth. 2005;52:1093–8.
129. Mahaffey KW, Lewis BE, Wildermann NM, et al. The anticoagulant therapy with bivalirudin to assist in the performance of percutaneous coronary intervention in patients with heparin induced thrombocytopenia (ATBAT) study: main results. J Invasive Cardiol. 2003;15:611–6.
130. Lincoff AM, Bittl JA, Harrington RA, et al. Bivalirudin and provisional glycoprotein IIb/IIIa blockade compared with heparin and planned glycoprotein IIb/IIIa blockade during percutaneous coronary intervention: REPLACE-2 randomized trial. JAMA. 2003;289:853–63.
131. Mehran R, Lansky AJ, Witzenbichler B, et al. Bivalirudin in patients undergoing primary angioplasty for acute myocardial infarction (HORIZONS-AMI): 1-year results of a randomised controlled trial. Lancet. 2009;374:1149–59.
132. Stone GW, Witzenbichler B, Guagliumi G, et al. Heparin plus a glycoprotein IIb/IIIa inhibitor versus bivalirudin monotherapy and paclitaxel-eluting stents versus bare-metal stents in acute myocardial infarction (HORIZONS-AMI): final 3-year results from a multicentre, randomised controlled trial. Lancet. 2011;377:2193–204.
133. Dangas GD, Claessen BE, Mehran R, Brener S, et al. Clinical outcomes following stent thrombosis occurring in-hospital versus out-of-hospital: results from the HORIZONS-AMI (Harmonizing Outcomes with Revascularization and Stents in Acute Myocardial Infarction) trial. J Am Coll Cardiol. 2012;59:1752–9.
134. Dangas G, Mehran R, Guagliumi G, et al. Role of clopidogrel loading dose in patients with ST-segment elevation myocardial infarction undergoing primary angioplasty: results from the HORIZONS-AMI (harmonizing outcomes with revascularization and stents in acute myocardial infarction) trial. J Am Coll Cardiol. 2009;54:1438–46.
135. Boneu B, Necciari J, Cariou R, et al. Pharmacokinetics and tolerance of the natural pentasaccharide (SR90107/Org31540)

with high affinity to antithrombin III in man. Thromb Haemost. 1995;74:1468–73.

136. Donat F, Duret JP, Santoni A, et al. The pharmacokinetics of fondaparinux sodium in healthy volunteers. Clin Pharmacokinet. 2002;41:1–9.

137. Lieu C, Shi J, Donat F, et al. Fondaparinux sodium is not metabolised in mammalian liver fractions and does not inhibit cytochrome P450-mediated metabolism of concomitant drugs. Clin Pharmacokinet. 2002;41:19–26.

138. Bassand JP, Hamm CW, Ardissino D, et al. Guidelines for the diagnosis and treatment of non-ST-segment elevation acute coronary syndromes. Eur Heart J. 2007;28:1598–660.

139. Paolucci F, Clavies MC, Donat F, et al. Fondaparinux sodium mechanism of action: identification of specific binding to purified and human plasma-derived proteins. Clin Pharmacokinet. 2002;41:11–8.

140. Savi P, Chong BH, Greinacher A, et al. Effect of fondaparinux on platelet activation in the presence of heparin-dependent antibodies: a blinded comparative multicenter study with unfractionated heparin. Blood. 2005;105:139–44.

141. Kuo KH, Kovacs MJ. Fondaparinux: a potential new therapy for HIT. Hematology. 2005;10:271–5.

142. Parody R, Oliver A, Souto JC, et al. Fondaparinux (ARIXTRA) as an alternative antithrombotic prophylaxis when there is hypersensitivity to low molecular weight and unfractionated heparins. Haematologica. 2003;88:ECR32.

143. Matziolis G, Perka C, Disch A, et al. Effects of fondaparinux compared with dalteparin, enoxaparin and unfractionated heparin on human osteoblasts. Calcif Tissue Int. 2003;73:370–9.

144. Lagrange F, Vergnes C, Brun JL, et al. Absence of placental transfer of pentasaccharide (Fondaparinux, Arixtra) in the dually perfused human cotyledon in vitro. Thromb Haemost. 2002;87:831–5.

145. Simoons ML, Bobbink IW, Boland J, et al. A dose-finding study of fondaparinux in patients with non-ST-segment elevation acute coronary syndromes: the Pentasaccharide in Unstable Angina (PENTUA) Study. J Am Coll Cardiol. 2004;43:2183–90.

146. Bijsterveld NR, Moons AH, Boekholdt SM, et al. Ability of recombinant factor VIIa to reverse the anticoagulant effect of the pentasaccharide fondaparinux in healthy volunteers. Circulation. 2002;106:2550–4.

147. Yusuf S, Mehta SR, Chrolavicius S, et al. Comparison of fondaparinux and enoxaparin in acute coronary syndromes. N Engl J Med. 2006;354:1464–76.

148. Steg PG, Mehta S, Jolly S, et al. Fondaparinux with UnfracTionated heparin dUring Revascularization in Acute coronary syndromes (FUTURA/OASIS 8): a randomized trial of intravenous

unfractionated heparin during percutaneous coronary intervention in patients with non-ST-segment elevation acute coronary syndromes initially treated with fondaparinux. Am Heart J. 2010;160:1029–34.

149. Yusuf S, Mehta SR, Chrolavicius S, et al. Effects of fondaparinux on mortality and reinfarction in patients with acute ST-segment elevation myocardial infarction: the OASIS-6 randomized trial. JAMA. 2006;295:1519–30.

150. Hinder M, Frick A, Jordaan P, et al. Direct and rapid inhibition of factor Xa by otamixaban: a pharmacokinetic and pharmacodynamic investigation in patients with coronary artery disease. Clin Pharmacol Ther. 2006;80:691–702.

151. Cohen M, Bhatt DL, Alexander JH, et al. Randomized, double-blind, dose-ranging study of otamixaban, a novel, parenteral, short-acting direct factor Xa inhibitor, in percutaneous coronary intervention: the SEPIA-PCI trial. Circulation. 2007;115:2642–51.

152. Sabatine MS, Antman EM, Widimsky P, et al. Otamixaban for the treatment of patients with non-ST-elevation acute coronary syndromes (SEPIA-ACS1 TIMI 42): a randomised, double-blind, active-controlled, phase 2 trial. Lancet. 2009;374:787–95.

153. Steg PG, Mehta SR, Pollack Jr CV, et al. Design and rationale of the treatment of acute coronary syndromes with otamixaban trial: a double-blind triple-dummy 2-stage randomized trial comparing otamixaban to unfractionated heparin and eptifibatide in non-ST-segment elevation acute coronary syndromes with a planned early invasive strategy. Am Heart J. 2012;164:817–24.

154. Angiolillo DJ, Ueno M, Goto S. Basic principles of platelet biology and clinical implications. Circ J. 2010;74:597 607.

155. Eikelboom JW, Weitz JI, Budaj A, et al. Clopidogrel does not suppress blood markers of coagulation activation in aspirin-treated patients with non-ST-elevation acute coronary syndromes. Eur Heart J. 2002;23:1771–9.

156. Hurlen M, Abdelnoor M, Smith P, et al. Warfarin, aspirin, or both after myocardial infarction. N Engl J Med. 2002;347:969–74.

157. Herlitz J, Holm J, Peterson M, et al. Effect of fixed low-dose warfarin added to aspirin in the long term after acute myocardial infarction: the LoWASA Study. Eur Heart J. 2004;25:232–9.

158. Orford JL, Fasseas P, Melby S, et al. Safety and efficacy of aspirin, clopidogrel, and warfarin after coronary stent placement in patients with an indication for anticoagulation. Am Heart J. 2004;1473:463–7.

159. Karjalainen PP, Porela P, Ylitalo A, et al. Safety and efficacy of combined antiplatelet-warfarin therapy after coronary stenting. Eur Heart J. 2007;286:726–32.

160. Khurram Z, Chou E, Minutello R, et al. Combination therapy with aspirin, clopidogrel and warfarin following coronary stenting is associated with a significant risk of bleeding. J Invasive Cardiol. 2006;184:162–4.

161. Becker RC. Antithrombotic therapy after myocardial infarction. N Engl J Med. 2002;347:1019–22.
162. Connolly SJ, Ezekowitz MD, Yusuf S, et al. Dabigatran versus warfarin in patients with atrial fibrillation. N Engl J Med. 2009;361:1139–51.
163. Patel MR, Mahaffey KW, Garg J, et al. Rivaroxaban versus warfarin in nonvalvular atrial fibrillation. N Engl J Med. 2011;365:883–9.
164. Connolly SJ, Eikelboom J, Joyner C, et al. Apixaban in patients with atrial fibrillation. N Engl J Med. 2011;364:806–17.
165. Stangier J, Rathgen K, Stähle H, et al. Influence of renal impairment on the pharmacokinetics and pharmacodynamics of oral dabigatran etexilate: an open-label, parallel-group, single-centre study. Clin Pharmacokinet. 2010;49:259–68.
166. Schulman S, Crowther MA. How I treat with anticoagulants in 2012: new and old anticoagulants, and when and how to switch. Blood. 2012;119:3016–23.
167. Spyropoulos AC, Douketis JD. How I treat anticoagulated patients undergoing an elective procedure or surgery. Blood. 2012;120:2954–62.
168. Wallentin L, Wilcox RG, Weaver WD, et al. ESTEEM Investigators. Oral ximelagatran for secondary prophylaxis after myocardial infarction: the ESTEEM randomised controlled trial. Lancet. 2003;362:789–97.
169. Sorbera LA, Bozzo J, Castaner J. Dabigatran/dabigatran etexilate. Drugs Fut. 2005;30:877–85.
170. Stangier J, Eriksson BI, Dahl OE, et al. Pharmacokinetic profile of the oral direct thrombin inhibitor dabigatran etexilate in healthy volunteers and patients undergoing total hip replacement. J Clin Pharmacol. 2005;45:555–63.
171. Eriksson BI, Dahl OE, Ahnfelt L, et al. Dose escalating safety study of a new oral direct thrombin inhibitor, dabigatran etexilate, in patients undergoing total hip replacement: BISTRO I. J Thromb Haemost. 2004;2:1573–80.
172. De Caterina R, Husted S, Wallentin L. New oral anticoagulants in atrial fibrillation and acute coronary syndromes: ESC Working Group on Thrombosis-Task Force on Anticoagulants in Heart Disease position paper. J Am Coll Cardiol. 2012;59:1413–25.
173. Eerenberg ES, Kamphuisen PW, Sijpkens MK, et al. Reversal of rivaroxaban and dabigatran by prothrombin complex concentrate: a randomized, placebo-controlled, crossover study in healthy subjects. Circulation. 2011;124:1573–9.
174. Oldgren J, Budaj A, Granger CB, et al. Dabigatran vs. placebo in patients with acute coronary syndromes on dual antiplatelet therapy: a randomized, double-blind, phase II trial. Eur Heart J. 2011;32:2781–9.
175. Jiang J, Hu Y, Zhang J, et al. Safety, pharmacokinetics and pharmacodynamics of single doses of rivaroxaban -an oral, direct

factor Xa inhibitor- in elderly Chinese subjects. Thromb Haemost. 2010;103:234–41.

176. Steg PG, Mehta SR, Jukema JW, et al. RUBY-1: a randomized, double-blind, placebo-controlled trial of the safety and tolerability of the novel oral factor Xa inhibitor darexaban (YM150) following acute coronary syndrome. Eur Heart J. 2011;32:2541–54.

177. Alexander JH, Becker RC, Bhatt DL, et al. Apixaban, an oral, direct, selective factor Xa inhibitor, in combination with antiplatelet therapy after acute coronary syndrome: results of the Apixaban for Prevention of Acute Ischemic and Safety Events (APPRAISE) trial. Circulation. 2009;119:2877–85.

178. Alexander JH, Lopes RD, James S, et al. The APPRAISE 2 Investigators. Apixaban with antiplatelet therapy after acute coronary syndrome. N Engl J Med. 2011;365:699–708.

179. Mega JL, Braunwald E, Mohanavelu S, et al. Rivaroxaban versus placebo in patients with acute coronary syndromes (ATLAS ACSTIMI 46): a randomised, double-blind, phase II trial. Lancet. 2009;374:29–38.

180. Gibson CM, Mega JL, Burton P, et al. Rationale and design of the Anti-Xa therapy to lower cardiovascular events in addition to standard therapy in subjects with acute coronary syndrome-thrombolysis in myocardial infarction 51 (ATLAS-ACS 2 TIMI 51) trial: a randomized, double-blind, placebo-controlled study to evaluate the efficacy and safety of rivaroxaban in subjects with acute coronary syndrome. Am Heart J. 2011;161:815–21.

181. Mega JL, Braunwald E, Wiviott SD, et al. Rivaroxaban in patients with a recent acute coronary syndrome. N Engl J Med. 2012;366:9–19.

182. Becker RC, Rusconi C, Sullenger B. Nucleic acid aptamers in therapeutic anticoagulation. Technology, development, and clinical application. Thromb Haemost. 2005;93:1014–20.

183. Becker RC, Povsic TJ, Cohen MG, et al. Nucleic acid aptamers as antithrombotic agents: opportunities in extracellular therapeutics. Thromb Haemost. 2010;103:586–95.

184. Povsic T, Sullenger B, Zelenkofske S, et al. Translating nucleic acid aptamers to antithrombotic drugs in cardiovascular medicine. J Cardiovasc Transl Res. 2011;3:704–16.

185. Povsic TJ, Cohen MG, Chan MY, et al. Dose selection for a direct and selective factor IXa inhibitor and its complementary reversal agent: translating pharmacokinetic and pharmacodynamic properties of the REG1 system to clinical trial design. J Thromb Thrombolysis. 2011;32:21–31.

186. Dyke CK, Steinhubl SR, Kleiman NS, et al. First-in-human experience of an antidote-controlled anticoagulant using RNA aptamer technology: a phase 1a pharmacodynamic evaluation of a drug-antidote pair for the controlled regulation of factor IXa activity. Circulation. 2006;114:2490–7.

187. Chan MY, Cohen MG, Dyke CK, et al. Phase 1b randomized study of antidote-controlled modulation of factor IXa activity in patients with stable coronary artery disease. Circulation. 2008;117:2865–74.
188. Chan MY, Rusconi CP, Alexander JH, et al. A randomized, repeat-dose, pharmacodynamic and safety study of an antidotecontrolled factor IXa inhibitor. J Thromb Haemost. 2008;6:789–96.
189. Cohen MG, Purdy DA, Rossi JS, et al. First clinical application of an actively reversible direct factor IXa inhibitor as an anticoagulation strategy in patients undergoing percutaneous intervention. Circulation. 2010;122:614–22.
190. Povsic TJ, Cohen MG, Mehran R, et al. A randomized, partially-blinded, multicenter, activecontrolled, dose-ranging study assessing the safety, efficacy, and pharmacodynamics of the REG1 anticoagulation system in patients with acute coronary syndromes: design and rationale of the RADAR phase IIb trial. Am Heart J. 2011;161:261–8.
191. Povsic TJ, Wargin WA, Alexander JH, et al. Pegnivacogin results in near complete FIX inhibition in acute coronary syndrome patients: RADAR pharmacokinetic and pharmacodynamic substudy. Eur Heart J. 2011;32:2412–9.
192. Esmon CT. Crosstalk between inflammation and thrombosis. Maturitas. 2004;47:305–14.
193. Coughlin SR. Protease-activated receptors in haemostasis, thrombosis and vascular biology. J Thromb Haemost. 2005;3:1800–14.
194. Ruf W, Dorfleutner A, Riewald M. Specificity of coagulation factor signalling. J Thromb Haemost. 2003;1:1495–503.
195. Morrow DA, Braunwald E, Bonaca MP, et al. Vorapaxar in the secondary prevention of atherothrombotic events. N Engl J Med. 2012;366:1404–13.
196. Tricoci P, Huang Z, Held C, et al. Thrombin-receptor antagonist vorapaxar in acute coronary syndromes. N Engl J Med. 2012;366:20–33.
197. Collin N, Assumpção TC, Mizurini DM, et al. Lufaxin, a Novel Factor Xa Inhibitor From the Salivary Gland of the Sand Fly Lutzomyia longipalpis Blocks Protease-Activated Receptor 2 Activation and Inhibits Inflammation and Thrombosis In Vivo. Arterioscler Thromb Vasc Biol. 2012;32:2185–98.

Chapter 4
Secondary Prevention in ACS: The Role of Novel Oral Anticoagulants

Hyun-Jae Kang and Matthew T. Roe

Brief Review of Current Antithrombotic Treatment Options and Recommendations from Guidelines for Secondary Prevention of ACS

For the contemporary management of acute coronary syndromes, antiplatelet therapy with aspirin and a $P2Y_{12}$ inhibitor is the benchmark antithrombotic strategy for secondary prevention after ACS. However, considering that thrombosis is one of the key steps in the pathogenesis of ACS, long term anticoagulation has the potential to be considered as a therapeutic option, in addition to dual anti-platelet therapy, to prevent recurrent ischemic events.

H.-J. Kang, MD, PhD
Division of Cardiology, Duke Clinical Research Institute,
2400 Pratt St., Rm. 7463, Durham, NC 27705, USA
e-mail: nowkang@snu.ac.kr

M.T. Roe, MD, MHS (✉)
Division of Cardiology, Duke Clinical Research Institute,
2400 Pratt St., Rm. 7035, Durham, NC 27705, USA
e-mail: matthew.roe@duke.edu

P. Avanzas, P. Clemmensen (eds.), *Pharmacological Treatment*
of Acute Coronary Syndromes, Current Cardiovascular Therapy,
DOI 10.1007/978-1-4471-5424-2_4,
© Springer-Verlag London 2014

Parenteral or subcutaneous anticoagulants are effective for reducing cardiovascular events during acute phase of acute coronary syndrome and recommended for all ACS patients without contraindications [1–6]. Anticoagulant options during the acute treatment phase of ACS include unfractionated heparin, low molecular weight heparin, fondaparinux, and bivalirudin. These agents are recommended to be used together with dual anti-platelet therapy during the index ACS hospitalization before and during invasive procedures such as angiography, percutaneous coronary intervention (PCI), and coronary artery bypass grafting (CABG). While treatment with low molecular weight heparins including enoxaparin and dalteparin for up to a few months after ACS has been studied in previous trials, logistical and cost considerations have limited the use of these anticoagulants in the post-discharge setting [7–9].

Warfarin, an oral anticoagulant, has been evaluated for long term secondary prevention of ACS during the past two decades. Long term anticoagulation with warfarin plus aspirin was more effective for reduction of cardiovascular events than aspirin alone in secondary prevention of ACS, but did not reduce mortality [10]. However, long term anticoagulation with warfarin, in conjunction with aspirin, was associated with a significant increased risk of bleeding. "Triple therapy" with warfarin and dual antiplatelet therapy (aspirin + clopidogrel) is associated with an even higher bleeding risk than warfarin + aspirin, but this combination of medications has not been evaluated in a large enough trial to determine if there is an efficacy advantage that could counterbalance the high bleeding risk [11]. Consequently, routine anticoagulation with warfarin after ACS, in addition to dual anti-platelet therapy, is not recommended.

Long term treatment with warfarin is only recommended for ACS patients who have indications for long term anticoagulation such as atrial fibrillation with at least a moderately high thromboembolic risk, presence of a mechanical valve prosthesis, or a concomitant venous thrombotic disorder such as a deep venous thrombosis [1–6].

The introduction of new, potent $P2Y_{12}$ inhibitors, prasugrel and ticagrelor, in the last 5 years has further established the role of dual anti-platelet therapy for the secondary prevention of ACS as both of these agents have been shown to be superior compared with aspirin and clopidogrel [12]. Current practice guidelines endorse both prasugrel and ticagrelor, in combination with aspirin, for the secondary prevention of high risk ACS patients [2–6].

Novel Oral Anti-coagulants for the Treatment of Patients with Recent ACS

There are two classes of new oral anticoagulants; direct factor Xa inhibitors and direct thrombin inhibitors. New oral anticoagulants have more predictable pharmacokinetic and pharmacodynamic characteristics than warfarin that facilitates their use without routine monitoring of anticoagulation activities at fixed doses. While these novel oral anticoagulants have shown superior efficacy and safety profiles in comparison with warfarin for patients with atrial fibrillation [13–15], the results with these agents for the secondary prevention of ACS have been more variable. Although the new parenteral direct factor Xa inhibitor otamixaban was evaluated for acute phase of treatment of ACS [16] in a dose-finding study and is currently being evaluated in a large phase III trial, otamixaban will not be discussed in this manuscript since it is a parenteral anticoagulant.

Direct Thrombin Inhibitors

Ximelagatran

In the 'efficacy and safety of the oral direct thrombin inhibitor ximelagatran in patients with recent myocardial damage (ESTEEM)' trial [17], ximelagatran was with background aspirin therapy was evaluated in medically treated ACS patients within 14 days of initial presentation. Ximelagatran significantly reduced the risk of the primary efficacy composite end point of death, myocardial infarction and recurrent severe ischemia compared with placebo (12.7 % vs. 16.3 %, hazard ratio [HR] 0.76; 95 % confidence interval [CI] 0.59–0.98, p=0.036). There was no dose response relationship among ximelagatran dosing groups regarding cardiovascular event reduction and there was no significant increase in major bleeding in the ximelagatran groups (1.8 % vs. 0.9 %, HR 1.97, 95 % CI 0.80–4.84). Despite these intriguing findings in this dose-ranging trial, ximelagatran was development was halted due to liver toxicity.

Dabigatran

Dabigatran is a pro-drug which has direct thrombin inhibitor activity with a serum half-life of 12–17 h and is excreted renally. The phase II Dose Finding Study for Dabigatran Etexilate in Patients with Acute Coronary Syndrome (REDEEM) trial evaluated the safety of dabigatran in stabilized 1,861 ACS patients who were enrolled within 14 days after index ACS event and treated with dual antiplatelet therapy. Dabigatran was associated with a dose-dependent increase in the primary safety endpoint of ISTH major or clinically relevant minor bleeding during the 6 month treatment period [18]. There was a dose-dependent increase of bleeding with dabigatran (twice daily at dose of 50 mg: 3.5 %, 75 mg: 4.3 %, 110 mg: 7.9 %, and 150 mg: 7.8 % vs. placebo: 2.2 %, p<0.001 for trend among dabigatran groups) during 6 months follow up. However there was no significant difference in the composite efficacy endpoint of cardiovascular death, non-fatal myocardial infarction, or non-haemorrhagic stroke between groups (dabigatran 50 mg: 4.6 %, 75 mg: 4.9 %, 110 mg: 3.0 %, 150 mg: 3.5 % vs. placebo: 3.8 %). However the two high dose groups (110, 150 mg) showed numerically lower event rates compared with the two low dose groups. All dabigatran doses were associated with significant further decreases of D-dimer level without dose-response relationship during first 4 weeks after treatment compared with placebo. Based upon these findings, further development of dabigatran for an ACS indication has not been pursued.

Direct Factor Xa Inhibitors

Darexaban

Darexaban is a direct factor Xa inhibitor with a terminal half-life of 14–18 h and equally gut and renal excretion. A randomized, double-blind, placebo-controlled trial of the safety and tolerability of the novel oral factor Xa inhibitor darexaban following acute coronary syndrome (RUBY-1) trial evaluated the safety of darexaban for secondary prevention of 1,279 high risk ACS patients who were enrolled within 7 days after index event and treated with dual antiplatelet therapy [19]. There was a dose-dependent increase of ISTH major and clinically relevant non-major bleeding event rates in the combined darexaban groups vs. placebo (pooled HR 2.275; 95 % CI 1.13–4.60, P = 0.022) (P = 0.009 for trend across darexaban dosing groups). The rate of all cause death, nonfatal myocardial infarction, nonfatal stroke, and severe recurrent ischemia was similar between the pooled darexaban groups vs. placebo (darexaban: 6.5 % vs. placebo: 5.2 %). Given these findings, darexaban has not been developed further for an ACS indication.

Apixaban

Apixaban is a direct factor Xa inhibitor with half-life of 12 h and predominantly eliminated by non-renal mechanisms. Apixaban for Prevention of Acute Ischemic and Safety Events (APPRAISE-1) trial was a phase II trial, which evaluated apixaban in stabilized recent ACS patients within 7 days with at least one risk factor for recurrent ischemic event [20]. There was a dose dependent increase of bleeding risk across the 4 dosing regimens of apixaban and the two higher dose groups with 10 mg twice daily or 20 mg once daily were discontinued prematurely because of excessive total bleeding. Apixaban 2.5 mg twice daily (HR 1.78; 95 % CI 0.91–3.48, P = 0.09) and 10 mg once daily (HR 2.45; 95 % CI 1.31–4.61, P = 0.005) also resulted in an increased risk of ISTH major or clinically relevant non-major bleeding. The increase in bleeding with the higher 2 doses of apixaban was more evident in patients taking clopidogrel. The two dosing groups, Apixaban 2.5 mg twice daily (HR 0.73; 95 % CI 0.44–1.19, P = 0.21) and 10 mg once daily (HR 0.61; 95 % CI 0.35–1.04, P = 0.07),were both associated with lower rates of the composite ischemic endpoint of cardiovascular death, myocardial infarction, severe recurrent ischemia, or ischemic stroke compared with placebo. These promising results led to a large, phase III trial for the ACS indication.

The efficacy of apixaban for the secondary prevention of ACS was evaluated in 7,392 stabilized recent, high risk ACS patients with 2 or more risk factors in the APPRAISE-2 trial [21]. This trial was terminated prematurely because of excessive increase in major bleeding events with apixaban, including a higher risk for intracranial hemorrhage. During an average follow-up period of 8 months, apixaban did not reduce the primary outcome of cardiovascular death, myocardial infarction, or ischemic stroke (apixaban: 7.5 % vs. placebo: 7.9 %, HR 0.95; 95 % CI 0.80–1.11, P = 0.51). Additionally, the risk of Thrombolysis in Myocardial Infarction (TIMI) major bleeding was more common in the apixaban group (1.3 %) compared with the placebo group (0.5 %, HR 2.59; 95 % CI 1.50–4.46, P = 0.001).

Rivaroxaban

Rivaroxaban is a direct factor Xa inhibitor with half-life of 5–7 h and eliminated by renal and gut excretion. In the phase II 'Anti-Xa Therapy to Lower cardiovascular events in addition to Aspirin with or without thienopyridine therapy in

Subjects with Acute Coronary Syndrome-Thrombolysis In Myocardial Infarction 46 (ATLASACS-1)' trial [22], rivaroxaban was evaluated in 3,491 stabilized recent ACS patients. The combined rivaroxaban dosing groups demonstrated a non-significant increase in the risk of the primary safety endpoint compared with placebo (composite of TIMI major, minor or requiring medical attention: 7.0 % vs. 5.6 %: p=0.10). There were dose dependent increases of bleeding (p<0.0001 for trend) with rivaroxaban treatment both with aspirin and aspirin+clopidogrel. An unexpected finding was that a reduced risk of the efficacy endpoint was demonstrated in the combined rivaroxaban groups (composite of death, myocardial infarction, or stroke: 3.9 % vs. 5.5 %: p=0.027). Additionally, a significant reduction in the net clinical benefit (composite of death, myocardial infarction, stroke, severe recurrent ischemia requiring revascularisation, TIMI major bleeding, or TIMI minor bleeding) was demonstrated with rivaroxaban compared with placebo only in patients treated with aspirin monotherapy (HR 0.56; 95 % CI 0.35–0.88), but not in the entire cohort (HR 0.99; 95 % CI0.76–1.29) and not in patients treated with dual antiplatelet therapy (HR 1.29; 95 % CI 0.93–1.81).. For the low dosing groups (2.5 mg or 5 mg of rivaroxaban twice daily), the net clinical benefit with rivaroxaban compared with placebo showed a potential signal for benefit with an HR of0.72 (0.46–1.12) in the entire cohort.

Based upon the ATLAS ACS-1 findings, the ALTAS ACS-2 trial was conducted in 15,526 stabilized recent ACS patients (within 7 days) who were treated with twice daily doses of either 2.5 mg or 5 mg of rivaroxaban vs. placebo for a mean of 13 months [23]. The combined rivaroxaban groups were shown to have a significant reduction in the risk of the primary composite efficacy end point of cardiovascular death, myocardial infarction, or stroke compared with placebo (8.9 % vs. 10.7 %, HR 0.84; 95 % CI 0.74–0.96, P=0.008), with similar results both the twice daily 2.5 mg dose (9.1 % vs. 10.7 %, P=0.02,) and the twice daily 5 mg dose (8.8 % vs.

10.7 %, P = 0.03,). Unexpectedly, the twice daily 2.5 mg dose of rivaroxaban was associated with a significant reduction in the risk of cardiovascular death (2.7 % vs. 4.1 %, P = 0.002) and all-cause death (2.9 % vs. 4.5 %, P = 0.002). However, the combined rivaroxaban dosing groups were associated with increased rates of major bleeding not related to CABG (2.1 % vs. 0.6 %, P < 0.001,) and intracranial hemorrhage (0.6 % vs. 0.2 %, P = 0.009) compared with placebo. Currently, rivaroxaban is undergoing regulatory review in both Europe and the United States for an ACS indication.

Safety Data with the Use of Novel Oral Anticoagulants for the Treatment of Patients with Recent ACS

Across 7 trials with 5 different medications, new oral anticoagulants have shown a consistent dose response relationship for bleeding risks. In general, doses of new anticoagulants used for patients with atrial fibrillation were associated with excessive bleeding in ACS patients primarily due to the fact that oral anticoagulant was usually evaluated as adjunct to mono- or dual-antiplatelet therapy. In the APPRAISE-2 trial [21], the 5 mg twice daily dose of apixaban, which was same dose used in the ARISTOTLE trial for atrial fibrillation [14], resulted in excessive bleeding without concomitant efficacy benefit leading to premature trial termination. A dose response in bleeding risk was also observed in the ATLAS ACS-2 trial, despite using cumulative doses of rivaroxaban lower than those used in the ROCKET trial for atrial fibrillation (2.5, 5.0 mg twice daily vs. 15/20 mg once daily) [15, 23]. Interestingly, the higher dose of rivaroxaban showed no efficacy advantage compared with the lower dose of rivaroxaban that was associated with a significant reduction in the risk of mortality.

Concomitant antiplatelet therapy is also an important determinant for bleeding risk with new oral anticoagulants in the post-ACS setting. Increases in bleeding were more evident when oral anticoagulants were used with dual antiplatelet therapy than aspirin alone [20, 22, 24].

Balancing Ischemic Vs. Bleeding Risks

The clinical usefulness for the adjunctive use of new oral anticoagulants should be discussed in terms of net clinical benefit. To justify the use of anticoagulants, absolute clinical benefit from ischemic event reduction should outweigh the expected increase in bleeding events. We already have noticed similar trade-off between ischemic event reduction and increase in bleeding with prasugrel and ticagrelor vs. clopidogrel in high risk ACS patients. For example, prasugrel prevented 19 ischemic events at the cost of 6 major TIMI non CABG bleeding during an average 14.5 months of treatment [12]. Ticagrelor prevented 22 ischemic events at the cost of 6 major TIMI non CABG bleeding during an average 9 months of treatment [25]. In comparison, the 2.5 mg twice daily dose of rivaroxaban prevented 16 major ischemic events at the cost of 12 major TIMI non CABG bleeding [26]. A recently published meta-analysis reported that new oral anticoagulants in the post ACS setting prevented 13 major ischemic event at the cost of 9 TIMI major bleeding [27]. Thus, the net clinical benefit with adjunctive oral anticoagulants dose not compare favourably with dual antiplatelet therapy and thus does not justify the routine use of new oral anticoagulants for the secondary prevention of ACS.

Nonetheless, further study of shorter durations of anticoagulation may be warranted as previous meta-analyses for the use of warfarin with aspirin in ACS patients showed that the greatest absolute net clinical benefit was observed during the first 3 months of therapy [10]. Shorter durations of treatment with new oral anticoagulants may improve the risk vs. benefit calculations for these agents in the post-ACS setting, but may not be attractive from a commercial standpoint for the pharmaceutical industry (Tables 4.1 and 4.2).

TABLE 4.1 Profiles of the clinical trials

	Phase of clinical trial	Number of patients	Duration of study	Dual antiplatelet	Treatments
ESTEEM [17]	II	1,883	6 months	0 %	Ximelagatran 24, 36, 48, 60 mg twice daily or placebo
REDEEM [18]	II	1,861	6 months	99 %	Dabigatran 50, 75, 110 or 150 mg twice daily or placebo
RUBY-1 [19]	II	1,279	6 months	95 %	Darexaban 5, 15, 30 mg twice daily, 10, 30, 60 mg once daily or placebo
APPRAISE-1 [20]	II	1,715	6 months (10 mg twice daily and 20 mg once daily: terminated early)	76 %	Apixaban 2.5, 10 mg twice daily, 10, 20 mg once daily or placebo
APPRAISE-2 [21]	III	7,392	8 months (prematurely terminated)	81 %	Apixaban 5 mg twice daily or placebo
ATLAS ACS-1 TIMI46 [22]	II	3,491	6 months	75 %	Rivaroxaban 2.5, 5, 10 mg twice daily or 5, 10, 20 mg once daily with aspirin, or rivaroxaban 2.5, 5, 7.5, 10 mg twice daily or 5, 10, 15, 20 mg once daily with dual antiplatelet or placebo
ATLAS ACS-2 TIMI51 [23]	III	15,526	13 months	93 %	Rivaroxaban 2.5 or 5 mg twice daily or placebo

TABLE 4.2 Key results of the clinical trials

	Efficacy endpoint (anticoagulant vs. placebo)	All cause death (anticoagulant vs. placebo)	Bleeding endpoint (anticoagulant vs. placebo)
ESTEEM [17]	composite of all cause death, non-fatal myocardial infarction, and severe recurrent ischemia=12.7 % (24, 36, 48, 60 mg: 11.7 %, 13.5 %, 11.6 %, 12.7 %) vs. 16.3 %	1.4 % (all) vs. 4.1 %	ISTH major bleeding: 1.8 % (1.9 %, 0.7 %, 3.2 % 1.5 %) vs. 0.9 %
REDEEM [18]	composite of cardiovascular death, non-fatal myocardial infarction, and non-hemorrhagic stroke = 50, 75, 110, 150 mg: 4.6 %, 4.9 %, 3.0 %, 3.5 % vs. 3.8 %	2.1 % (all) vs. 3.8 %	ISTH major or clinically relevant minor bleeding: 1.1 % (3.5 %, 4.3 %, 7.9 %, 7.8 %) vs. 2.2 %
RUBY-1 [19]	composite of all-cause death, nonfatal myocardial infarction, non-fatal stroke, and severe recurrent ischemia=5.6 % (5, 15, 30 mg twice daily, 10, 30, 60 mg once daily; 3.8 %, 6.3 %, 5.9 %, 3.8 %, 6.4 %, 7.8 %) vs. 4.4 %	0.7 % (all) vs. 0.6 %	ISTH major or clinically relevant minor bleeding =5.7 %, 6.3 %, 9.8 %, 5.0 %, 5.1 %, 6.5 % vs. 2.8 %
APPRAISE-1 [20]	composite of cardiovascular death, MI, severe recurrent ischemia, or ischemic stroke = 2.5 mg twice daily, 10 mg once daily: 7.6 %, 6.0 % vs. 8.7 %	2.5 mg twice daily, 10 mg once daily: 3.5 %, 1.6 % vs. 2.0 %	ISTH major or clinically relevant minor bleeding =2.5 mg twice daily, 10 mg once daily, 10 mg twice daily, 20 mg once daily: 5.0 %, 5.6 %, 7.8 %, 7.3 % vs. 0.8 %

(continued)

TABLE 4.2 (continued)

	Efficacy endpoint (anticoagulant vs. placebo)	All cause death (anticoagulant vs. placebo)	Bleeding endpoint (anticoagulant vs. placebo)
APPRAISE-2 [21]	Composite of cardiovascular death, myocardial infarction, or ischemic stroke = 7.5 % vs. 7.9 %	4.2 % vs. 3.9 %	TIMI major bleeding = 1.3 % vs. 0.5 %
ATLAS ACS-1 TIMI46 [22]	the time to the first episode of death, myocardial infarction, stroke, or severe recurrent ischemia requiring revascularization (Kaplan Meier event rate) = 2.5, 5, 10 mg twice daily or 5, 10, 20 mg once daily; 5.3 %, 4.4 %, 6.5 %, 8.7 %, 5.3 %, 5.2 % vs. 7.0 %	Not available	Clinically significant bleeding (TIMI major, TIMI minor, or requiring medical attention) = 2.5, 5, 10 twice daily or 5, 10, 20 mg once daily; 4.8 %, 11.0 %, 14.6 %, 7.4 %, 10.8 %, 16.0 % vs. 3.3 %
ATLAS ACS-2 TIMI51 [23]	Composite of cardiovascular death, myocardial infarction, or stroke = 8.9 % (2.5 , 5 mg twice daily:9.1 %, 8.8 %) vs. 10.7 %	3.7 % (2.5, 5 mg: 2.9 %, 4.4 %) vs. 4.5 %	TIMI major non-CABG bleeding: 2.1 % (1.8 %, 2.4 %) vs. 0.6 %

- ISTH: International Society of Thrombosis and Haemostasis

- ISTH major bleeding: fatal bleeding; clinically overt bleeding associated with a fall in haemoglobin of at least 20 g/L or leading to transfusion of two or more units of whole blood or erythrocytes; bleeding in areas of special concern, such as intracranial, intraspinal, intraocular, retroperitoneal, pericardial, or atraumatic intra-articular bleeding

- Clinically relevant minor bleeding: a clinically overt bleed that did not meet the criteria for major bleed but prompted a clinical response

- TIMI: thrombolysis in myocardial infarction

- TIMI major bleeding: any intracranial bleeding, clinically overt signs of hemorrhage associated with a drop in hemoglobin of ≥ 5 g/dL or a ≥ 15 % absolute decrease in haematocrit, or fatal bleeding

- TIMI minor bleeding: clinically overt, resulting in hemoglobin drop of 3 to <5 g/dL or ≥ 10 % decrease in haematocrit, or no observed blood loss: ≥ 4 g/dL decrease in the haemoglobin concentration or ≥ 12 % decrease in haematocrit, any overt sign of hemorrhage requiring intervention or prompting evaluation, or leading to or prolonging hospitalization and does not meet criteria for a major bleeding event

Suggested Choices Based on Current Evidence

Regarding combination therapy, anticoagulation in conjunction with dual antiplatelet therapy is associated with an increased risk of bleeding and potential lower reduction in the risk of ischemic events compared with use of these agents with aspirin alone. Additionally, data regarding the use of new anticoagulants in conjunction with or in comparison with potent $P2Y_{12}$ inhibitors (prasugrel or ticagrelor) are not available. Thus, it is not recommended to use new oral anticoagulants together with or in place of prasugrel or ticagrelor. However, using new oral anticoagulants in ACS patients who have an indication for long term anticoagulation, in which warfarin is typically used, may be considered as a reasonable approach, but requires further study in dedicated trials that are just starting.

References

1. Anderson JL, Adams CD, et al. ACC/AHA 2007 guidelines for the management of patients with unstable angina/non ST-elevation myocardial infarction: a report of the American College of Cardiology/American Heart Association Task Force on Practice Guidelines (Writing Committee to Revise the 2002 Guidelines for the Management of Patients With Unstable Angina/Non ST-Elevation Myocardial Infarction): developed in collaboration with the American College of Emergency Physicians, the Society for Cardiovascular Angiography and Interventions, and the Society of Thoracic Surgeons: endorsed by the American Association of Cardiovascular and Pulmonary Rehabilitation and the Society for Academic Emergency Medicine. Circulation. 2007;116(7):e148–304.
2. Hamm CW, Bassand JP, et al. ESC Guidelines for the management of acute coronary syndromes in patients presenting without persistent ST-segment elevation: The Task Force for the management of acute coronary syndromes (ACS) in patients presenting without persistent ST-segment elevation of the European Society of Cardiology (ESC). Eur Heart. 2011;J32(23):2999–3054.
3. Jneid H, Anderson JL, et al. 2012 ACCF/AHA focused update of the guideline for the management of patients with unstable angina/non-ST-elevation myocardial infarction (updating the 2007 guideline and

replacing the 2011 focused update): a report of the American College of Cardiology Foundation/American Heart Association Task Force on Practice Guidelines. J Am Coll Cardiol. 2012;60(7):645–81.

4. Jneid H, Anderson JL, et al. 2012 ACCF/AHA focused update of the guideline for the management of patients with unstable angina/ Non-ST-elevation myocardial infarction (updating the 2007 guideline and replacing the 2011 focused update): a report of the American College of Cardiology Foundation/American Heart Association Task Force on practice guidelines. Circulation. 2012;126(7):875–910.

5. O'Gara PT, Kushner FG, et al. 2013 ACCF/AHA guideline for the management of ST-elevation myocardial infarction: a report of the American College of Cardiology Foundation/American Heart Association Task Force on Practice Guidelines. Circulation. 2013;127(4):e362–425.

6. Steg PG, James SK, et al. ESC Guidelines for the management of acute myocardial infarction in patients presenting with ST-segment elevation. Eur Heart. 2012;J33(20):2569–619.

7. Low-molecular-weight heparin during instability in coronary artery disease, Fragmin during Instability in Coronary Artery Disease (FRISC) study group (1996) Lancet. 347(9001):561 8.

8. Long-term low-molecular-mass heparin in unstable coronary-artery disease: FRISC II prospective randomised multicentre study. FRagmin and Fast Revascularisation during InStability in Coronary artery disease Investigators (1999) Lancet. 354(9180):701–7.

9. Cohen M, Demers C, et al. Low-molecular-weight heparins in non-ST-segment elevation ischemia: the ESSENCE trial. Efficacy and Safety of Subcutaneous Enoxaparin versus intravenous unfractionated heparin, in non Q-wave Coronary Events. Am J Cardiol. 1998; 82(5B):19L–24.

10. Rothberg MB, Celestin C, et al. Warfarin plus aspirin after myocardial infarction or the acute coronary syndrome: meta-analysis with estimates of risk and benefit. Ann Intern Med. 2005;143(4):241–50.

11. Sorensen R, Hansen ML, et al. Risk of bleeding in patients with acute myocardial infarction treated with different combinations of aspirin, clopidogrel, and vitamin K antagonists in Denmark: a retrospective analysis of nationwide registry data. Lancet. 2009;374(9706): 1967–74.

12. Wiviott SD, Braunwald E, et al. Prasugrel versus clopidogrel in patients with acute coronary syndromes. N Engl J Med. 2007;357(20): 2001–15.

13. Connolly SJ, Ezekowitz MD, et al. Dabigatran versus warfarin in patients with atrial fibrillation. N Engl J Med. 2009;361(12): 1139–51.

14. Granger CB, Alexander JH, et al. Apixaban versus warfarin in patients with atrial fibrillation. N Engl J Med. 2011;365(11):981–92.

15. Patel MR, Mahaffey KW, et al. Rivaroxaban versus warfarin in non-valvular atrial fibrillation. N Engl J Med. 2011;365(10):883–91.
16. Sabatine MS, Antman EM, et al. Otamixaban for the treatment of patients with non-ST-elevation acute coronary syndromes (SEPIA-ACS1 TIMI 42): a randomised, double-blind, active-controlled, phase 2 trial. Lancet. 2009;374(9692):787–95.
17. Wallentin L, Wilcox RG, et al. Oral ximelagatran for secondary prophylaxis after myocardial infarction: the ESTEEM randomised controlled trial. Lancet. 2003;362(9386):789–97.
18. Oldgren J, Budaj A, et al. Dabigatran vs. placebo in patients with acute coronary syndromes on dual antiplatelet therapy: a randomized, double-blind, phase II trial. Eur Heart. 2011;J32(22):2781–9.
19. Steg PG, Mehta SR, et al. RUBY-1: a randomized, double-blind, placebo-controlled trial of the safety and tolerability of the novel oral factor Xa inhibitor darexaban (YM150) following acute coronary syndrome. Eur Heart. 2011;J32(20):2541–54.
20. Alexander JH, Becker RC, et al. Apixaban, an oral, direct, selective factor Xa inhibitor, in combination with antiplatelet therapy after acute coronary syndrome: results of the Apixaban for Prevention of Acute Ischemic and Safety Events (APPRAISE) trial. Circulation. 2009;119(22):2877–85.
21. Alexander JH, Lopes RD, et al. Apixaban with antiplatelet therapy after acute coronary syndrome. N Engl J Med. 2011;365(8):699–708.
22. Mega JL, Braunwald E, et al. Rivaroxaban versus placebo in patients with acute coronary syndromes (ATLAS ACS-TIMI 46): a randomised, double-blind, phase II trial. Lancet. 2009;374(9683): 29–38.
23. Mega JL, Braunwald E, et al. Rivaroxaban in patients with a recent acute coronary syndrome. N Engl J Med. 2012;366(1):9–19.
24. Oldgren J, Wallentin L, et al. New oral anticoagulants in addition to single or dual antiplatelet therapy after an acute coronary syndrome: a systematic review and meta-analysis. Eur Heart J. 2013;34: 1670–80.
25. Wallentin L, Becker RC, et al. Ticagrelor versus clopidogrel in patients with acute coronary syndromes. N Engl J Med. 2009; 361(11):1045–57.
26. Roe MT, Ohman EM. A new era in secondary prevention after acute coronary syndrome. N Engl J Med. 2012;366(1):85–7.
27. Komocsi A, Vorobcsuk A, et al. Use of new-generation oral anticoagulant agents in patients receiving antiplatelet therapy after an acute coronary syndrome: systematic review and meta-analysis of randomized controlled trials. Arch Intern Med. 2012;172(20): 1537–45.

Chapter 5
American Versus European Guidelines: Critical Appraisal

Gabriella Passacquale and Albert Ferro

Introduction

The American and European Societies of Cardiology have recently issued updated guidelines for the management of ST-elevation myocardial infarction (STEMI) [1, 2] and non-STEMI/unstable angina (NSTEMI/UA) [3, 4]. The distinction between these two clinical manifestations of acute coronary syndrome (ACS) was first introduced in the 1996 publication of the "*ACC/AHA Guidelines for the Management of Patients with Acute Myocardial Infarction*" [5], when the term ACS was used to describe an episode of cardiac discomfort/pain arising from atherosclerotic plaque disruption. Patients suffering an ACS were categorized into STEMI and NSTEMI/UA on the basis of electrocardiography (ECG), to distinguish between those with likely complete thrombotic occlusion of a coronary artery leading to ST-elevation (STEMI patients) and those with putatively incomplete coronary artery occlusion in whom raised markers of myocardial necrosis would further distinguish myocardial infarction without ST-elevation

G. Passacquale, MD, PhD (✉)

A. Ferro, BSc (Hons), MBBS, PhD, FRCP
Department of Clinical Pharmacology,
King's College London, London, UK
e-mail: gabriella.passacquale@kcl.ac.uk; albert.ferro@kcl.ac.uk

P. Avanzas, P. Clemmensen (eds.), *Pharmacological Treatment*   139
of Acute Coronary Syndromes, Current Cardiovascular Therapy,
DOI 10.1007/978-1-4471-5424-2_5,
© Springer-Verlag London 2014

(NSTEMI) from UA. Almost concomitantly, the European Society of Cardiology (ESC) published the guidelines for "*Acute myocardial infarction: pre-hospital and in-hospital management*" [6] where a similar distinction was made between STEMI and non-STEMI-ACS.

Until the late 1990s, recommendations for the management of the two distinct types of ACS were discussed within the same guidelines, since they overlap in many aspects of the pharmacological treatment adopted in the acute and post-acute phases, the main difference being the immediate need for a reperfusion strategy that only applies to patients with ST segment elevation on 12-lead ECG, this being diagnostic for myocardial necrosis which often progresses to the development of Q waves. It was with the publication of the 2000 American guidelines for NSTEMI/UA [7] (followed by the 2003 ESC recommendations for STEMI [8]) that the need to distinguish the management of STEMI and NSTEMI/UA was emphasized, as a result of important advances in both medical and interventional therapies coupled with a growing evidence base that these conditions were best managed in different ways.

From a historical prospective, it is evident that major changes have occurred in all aspects of ACS management. Indeed, the value of different biomarkers of cardiac necrosis (cardiac troponins, creatine kinase-MB fraction and myoglobin) and the application of imaging modalities for myocardial infarction (MI) diagnosis have evolved over the years, leading to three revisions of the criteria for MI over the last decade [9–11]. The development of novel fibrinolytic, anti-platelet and anti-coagulant drugs now allows a multi-targeted pharmacological approach to ACS, with the rationale that acting on multiple therapeutic targets will provide a more comprehensive and hence more effective treatment of cardiovascular thrombotic events. Important advances in medical treatments have been paralleled by rapid progress in invasive reperfusion techniques, namely percutaneous coronary intervention (PCI), leading to the formulation of guidelines specifically dedicated to PCI [12] and myocardial revascularization [13]. This chapter will provide an overview of the changes in medical therapies for ACS that have occurred in Europe and North America in the last decade, and these are summarized in Fig. 5.1, which illustrates important milestones in the evolution of pharmacological management of ACS and how these have led to the current clinical

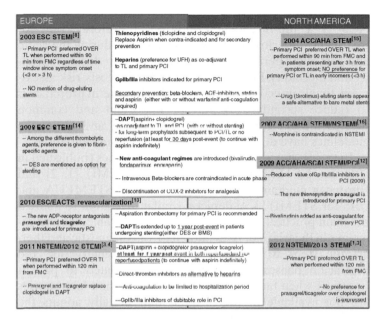

FIGURE 5.1 Evolution of ACS management in the last decade. Major changes have occurred over recent years in the management of ACS. In the middle the elements of common agreement are shown, whilst on the left and right hand sides the elements specific to ESC (*blue*) and ACC/AHA (*red*) respectively are displayed. *ESC* European Society of Cardiology, *ACC/AHA* American College of Cardiology/ American Heart Association, *EACTS* European Association of Cardio-Thoracic Surgery, *SCAI* Society for Cardiovascular Angiography and Interventions, *ACS* acute coronary syndrome, *BMS* bare metal stent, *DAPT* dual anti-platelet therapy, *FMC* first medical contact, *DES* drug-eluting stents, *PCI* percutaneous coronary intervention, *TL* thrombolysis, *UFH* unfractionated heparin

approach to management of STEMI and NSTEMI/UA –
including differences between the European and North
American guidelines.

Modern Management of Acute Coronary Syndrome: A General Overview

ACS is a life-threading condition, therefore "time-to-treatment" and close monitoring of patients during the acute and post-acute periods are crucial aspects in reducing mortality and morbidity. Prompt and accurate diagnosis, risk assessment, timely intervention and effective long-term prophylaxis to reduce secondary events are important and common themes around which both the American and European guidelines have developed their clinical recommendations.

In their last update, the American guidelines (published in 2011 for NSTEMI/UA and 2012 for STEMI) [1, 2] and European guidelines (issued in 2012 for NSTEMI/UA and 2013 for STEMI) [3, 4] depict a similar algorithm to address the main practical issues encountered by paramedics and clinicians in the triage of ACS patients, from diagnostic and therapeutic steps to be undertaken in the emergency and post-acute phases to logistical aspects related to patient transport when facilities such as catheterization laboratories are not available in the hospital that initially admits the patient. A theme that characterizes both guidelines is their emphasis on the need to implement diagnostic competencies and to promote regional networking in the pre-hospital setting, where first medical contact (FMC) occurs, so that clinical decisions are taken without delay. The definition of "timely" intervention since symptom onset has evolved over the years, as a result of a growing body of evidence demonstrating differences in time dependency of pharmacological and mechanical reperfusion therapies on main clinical outcomes [14, 15], with consequent impact on the choice of reperfusion strategy adopted in STEMI patients. Moreover, with the increasing availability of PCI that is gradually replacing the fibrinolytic approach to coronary reperfusion in many hospitals – albeit with important differences in its availability between the two continents [16] – the main question of how mechanical reperfusion therapy compares with a fibrinolytic strategy, with the object of defining whether optimal care can be offered to all patients regardless of whether they present to a PCI-capable or a PCI-incapable institution, has been a subject of much debate between Europe and North America. Similarly, in NSTEMI/UA patients, conservative versus invasive treatment, including timing for invasive diagnostic procedures (angiography) and subsequent coronary revascularization (when indicated), are important, and as yet unresolved, issues.

From a pharmacological prospective, a number of novel treatments have emerged in the latest versions of the ACS guidelines, mainly constituting drugs which reduce blood thrombogenicity. Indeed, the anti-platelet armamentarium has been enriched by the introduction of novel drugs with greater platelet inhibitory efficacy than the classical cyclooxygenase (COX) inhibitor aspirin and the second generation $P2Y_{12}$ ADP receptor antagonist clopidogrel (belonging to the thienopyridine drug class) [17, 18]. The third generation thienopyridine prasugrel and the reversible $P2Y_{12}$ antagonist ticagrelor have now been included in the contemporary American and European guidelines as part of dual anti-platelet therapy (DAPT), albeit with differences between the guidelines in their use and clinical indications (as specified later in this chapter). Anti-thrombotic therapy is central to the management of ACS in the emergency setting, where it acts as co-adjuvant both to reperfusion strategies and to conservative management (anti-ischaemic and analgesic therapy) to limit the propagation of arterial thrombus; similarly it is central to long-term prophylaxis for prevention of re-infarction as a result of atherosclerosis progression or re-stenosis of implanted stents. In the following paragraphs we will discuss important new developments in medical therapy as regards:

- Pre-hospital and emergency care;
- Reperfusion therapy: pharmacological versus mechanical;
- Anti-thrombotic regimes (anti-platelet and anti-coagulant drugs);
- Long-term therapy.

Pre-hospital and Emergency Care

The American and European guidelines each dedicate an extensive chapter to the emergency care of the ACS patient, including the pharmacological approach to analgesia, the use of anti-ischaemic (i.e. beta-blockers and nitrates) and anti-thrombotic drugs, and initiation of a pharmacological reperfusion strategy as appropriate with the main emphasis on the use of pre-hospital fibrinolysis (PHF). In all these areas major changes have occurred in the last decade, and with general consensus between Europe and North America. However, discrepancies are apparent between Europe and North America as regards the place that PHF holds in STEMI management, in part possibly because of differences in their health systems and availability of emergency PCI, but also because of differences in perceptions regarding the relative merits of pharmacological versus mechanical reperfusion strategies.

Analgesia

The 2004 ACC/AHA Task Forces for the management of STEMI recommended in their guidelines the use of morphine in all patients with ACS, regardless of whether the diagnosis was STEMI or NSTEMI/UA [19]. In the 2007 update [20], a distinction was made between the two clinical manifestations of the ACS on the basis of the CRUSADE study [21] that retrospectively analysed the safety of morphine (in terms of impact on in-hospital death, recurrent MI, congestive heart failure, and cardiogenic shock) in 57,039 patients with NSTEMI/UA; the results, published in 2005, demonstrated that the use of intravenous morphine, alone or in combination with nitroglycerin, increased mortality in this population. The hypotensive and cardio-respiratory depressive effects of morphine were advanced as possible explanations for this finding [21, 22]. The CRUSADE study led to a review of the level of evidence in support of the use of morphine for pain relief in patients with NSTEMI/UA, that from a recommended choice, although not supported by evidence-based literature and therefore classified as Class IC, became a reasonable option (Class IIa) and only in those cases where relief of symptoms is not achieved with nitroglycerin, as specified in the 2007 update for STEMI [20] and the 2009 updates for NSTEMI/UA of the ACC/AHA Task Force [12]. Unlike the cautious attitude manifested by the American guidelines, there is no mention of the CRUSADE study results in the consensus documents for STEMI or for NSTEMI/UA of the ESC, and morphine is indicated in the latest ESC recommendations for NSTEMI/UA among the initial therapeutic measures [3]. It is uncertain what the impact of morphine administration would be on clinical outcomes in patients who are treated with more modern strategies than those applicable at the time of the CRUSADE study, with much wider application of DAPT and reduced administration of beta-blockers in the acute phase as discussed below (in CRUSADE, about 40 and 80 % received DAPT and beta-blocker therapy respectively). Nevertheless, the CRUSADE study has brought to the attention of cardiologists worldwide the potential negative consequences of morphine administration in this subgroup of patients, in whom masking the symptoms of continued ischaemia without addressing the underlying cause might represent suboptimal treatment.

Both the 2007 ACC/AHA update for STEMI/NSTEMI [20] and the 2008 ESC guidelines for STEMI [23] have emphasized the potentially harmful effect of selective COX-2 inhibitors and indeed of non-steroidal anti-inflammatory drugs (NSAIDs) in general in ACS patients, given the increased cardiovascular risk associated with the use of these drugs as demonstrated in several epidemiological studies and retrospective analyses of randomized controlled trials (RCTs) [24–27]. Recommending the discontinuation of COX-2 inhibitors and NSAIDs at FMC, and advising against their use during in-hospital stay, are a feature in common of both the European and American guidelines in force currently.

Anti-ischaemic Drugs

The use of beta-blockers in the emergency care of ACS has a strong rationale in view of their pharmacological modulation of heart rate, systemic arterial pressure and myocardial contractility, in turn leading to a decrease in myocardial oxygen demand [23]. In the 2000 American Guidelines the early use of beta-blockers was highly recommended as a general approach to all patients presenting with STEMI, for their favourable effects in reduction of infarct size, re-infarction and occurrence of ventricular arrhythmias as reported by a number of clinical trials [28–30]. Uncertainty was expressed about the administration of beta-blockers via intravenous injection, and particularly in those patients undergoing fibrinolytic therapy, principally based on 2 randomized clinical trials and a post-hoc analysis of intravenous beta blockade that did not show benefit on mortality rate as compared with placebo [31–33]. The 2007 STEMI update further devalued the place of intravenous beta blockade in light of the evidence from the COMMIT trial that, in addition to a lack of favourable effect on mortality, showed an increase in the rate of cardiogenic shock in the group of patients receiving intravenous metoprolol compared with placebo, particularly in those with haemodynamic instability (regardless of whether the diagnosis was STEMI or NSTEMI) [34]. Therefore, intravenous beta-blockade is currently indicated only in cases of refractory tachyarrhythmia and hypertension and in patients without *"signs of heart failure, evidence of a low output state, increased risk for cardiogenic shock, or other relative contraindications to beta blockade (PR interval greater than 0.24 s, second- or third-degree heart block, active asthma, or reactive airway disease*)" (as reported in the 2007 ACC/AHA update of STEMI) [20]. Agreement can be seen in the ESC guidelines, where it is specified that initiation of oral beta blocker therapy requires stabilization of patients in the first instance [3]. Overall, the enthusiasm for early use of beta blockers in patients with MI (including STEMI and NSTEMI) that was promoted by both Europeans and Americans in their 2003–2004 guidelines has been moderated in more recent years by the growth of evidence demonstrating only a modest benefit of this class of drugs on mortality rate in stable patients [35]. On the other hand, the value of beta blockers in long-term prophylaxis is well established.

The anti-ischaemic value of nitrates has also been reappraised. Indeed, although useful in reducing coronary vasospasm, nitrates failed to show any benefit in reduction of infarct area or in mortality associated with MI, as demonstrated in the GISSI-3 [36] and ISIS-4 trials [37]. Therefore, routine use of nitrates in the initial phase of STEMI is not recommended, although it represents a useful therapeutic option for analgesia in NSTEMI/UA patients with ongoing pain. Table 5.1 shows the place of selected analgesic/anti-ischaemic medical

TABLE 5.1 Common analgesic and anti-ischaemic drugs in the initial management of ACS

Drugs	STEMI	NSTEMI
Morphine	First-line 4–8 mg i.v. + 2–8 mg i.v. every 5–10 min if needed	If not responding to nitrates 3.5 mg i.v or s.c.
Nitrates	[Limited usefulness] Sublingual or i.v. (caution if SBP <60 mmHg)	Sublingual or i.v. (caution if SBP <60 mmHg)
Beta-blockers	Oral: all pts with no contraindications Intravenous: for refractory Tachycardia and hypertension	Oral: for Tachycardia and hypertension without signs of HF

i.v. intravenous, *s.c.* subcutaneous, *HF* heart failure, *SBP* systolic blood pressure therapies in the acute management of ACS in accordance with current guidelines.

Pre-hospital Fibrinolysis

The strategy of initiating fibrinolysis in the pre-hospital setting was first described in the early 1990s [38], prior to the widespread development of invasive techniques to restore coronary patency (PCI) and when medical reperfusion therapy was the primary treatment for MI [39]. PHF only applies to STEMI patients, since in NSTEMI patients no benefit has ever been demonstrated for fibrinolysis, whereas the risks of this therapy are all too apparent in such patients [40]. By conferring a reduction in time to reperfusion from symptom onset, PHF reduces mortality rate associated with MI compared with in-hospital administration of thrombolytic therapy [38, 41, 42]. In a review of randomized controlled trials published between 1989 and 1999, Morrison et al. [42] reported that the beneficial effect of PHF on all cause mortality at 30 and 60 days was regardless of the lytic agent used (fibrin-specific alteplase (rtPA), anistreplase or urokinase). In 2000 a new fibrinolytic drug was launched, namely tenecteplase, a genetically engineered variant of alteplase that in the ASSENT-2 trial [43] showed similar efficacy with less bleeding complication than rtPA (likely because it is administered as a single bolus compared to dual injection for rtPA). Tenecteplase (co-administered with heparin, either low-molecular weight or unfractionated) was tested in the pre-hospital setting in the ASSENT-PLUS 3 trial in 2003 [44], and demonstrated safety and efficacy on the primary endpoints (mortality and re-infarction rates), with a greater favourable effect when enoxaparin (the low-molecular weight heparin used in this study) was co-administered. Given its ease of administration as a single bolus, and its higher specificity for fibrin compared with alteplase and retaplase [45] (thus accounting potentially for a lesser systemic fibrinolytic effect), tenecteplase is now regarded as a valuable thrombolytic option available in both the pre- and in-hospital settings.

A minor place is accorded to the use of the non-fibrin-specific streptokinase in contemporary recommendations. Indeed, in their most recent guidelines for STEMI, both Americans and Europeans express a preference for fibrin-specific drugs over streptokinase, a change to previous versions where no specific preferences were given to the choice of fibrinolytic agent other than considerations related to accessibility and cost. Nevertheless, streptokinase remains in widespread use because of its low cost, even though evidence of survival advantage provided by fibrin-specific drugs in comparison with streptokinase in STEMI has been available since the late 1990s with the publication of the GUSTO I and GUSTO III trials [46, 47]. Moreover, a study by Steg et al. [48] demonstrated that efficiency of fibrin-specific agents in clot dissolution is less dependent on time of administration than streptokinase.

Both the American and European guidelines have expressed a general consensus on the usefulness of PHF based on the rationale that earlier treatment promotes better survival rates, possibly because of greater efficacy of these drugs on early clots, which exhibit lesser fibrin cross-linking than older thrombi, with consequent better rates of coronary reperfusion and myocardial savage. Nevertheless, the use of PHF in North America and Europe is dramatically different, largely because of their distinct emergency system programmes [16, 17]. European countries have, by and large, developed more effective regional networking systems with telemetry (transmission of ECG from ambulances to local centres) and ambulances staffed with paramedics trained in ECG interpretation and MI treatment and/or physicians. However, with the now widespread application of primary PCI for coronary revascularization that is now regarded as first-line reperfusion strategy in all STEMI patients (assuming it can be performed in a timely fashion), and the fall into disuse of "facilitated" PCI (PCI performed immediately after administration of a full-dose of thrombolytic agent) which was found to increase in-hospital mortality compared to primary PCI (without fibrinolytic therapy) [49], the place of

PHF in the management of STEMI now seems far less clear (as further discussed below).

Reperfusion Strategy: Pharmacological Versus Mechanical

With the exclusion of those rural scenarios where fibrinolytic therapy is the only available therapeutic option (and where therefore PHF represents a valuable resource), the 2004 ACC/AHA Task Force stated that in STEMI patients who present within the first 3 h from symptom onset – and who otherwise have access to primary PCI – either a mechanical or medical reperfusion strategy achieved in a "timely" fashion (as specified in the following paragraphs) impact equally on survival. This was based on the results from the CAPTIM and PRAGUE-2 trials [50, 51]. The former reported no difference between PHF (performed with alteplase in combination with heparin and aspirin) and primary PCI on a 30-day composite end-point of mortality/non-fatal re-infarction and stroke, and even an advantage of PHF over mechanical reperfusion in the subgroup of patients presenting within 3 h from symptom onset. The latter showed comparable results for the two reperfusion strategies (in-hospital fibrinolysis with streptokinase in combination with aspirin, clopidogrel and fraxiparin versus primary PCI) in terms of all-cause mortality at 30 days when the analysis was restricted to early presenters (<3 h); in patients treated more than 3 h after symptom onset, fibrinolysis was associated with increased events compared with primary PCI (data are summarized in Table 5.2). The parallel 2003 ESC guidelines stated the superiority of PCI over fibrinolysis regardless of time since symptom onset. Indeed, the ESC writing committee concluded that the clinical evidence available at that time (including the CAPTIM, PRAGUE-2 and DANAMI-2 trials) [14, 50, 51] were not conclusive of equal efficacy of the two reperfusion strategies on clinical outcomes, including in patients presenting early. Specifically, the CAPTIM study actually compared primary PCI with a strategy of PHF followed by patient transport to an interventional centre for rescue PCI (that was performed in 25 % of patients assigned to PHF); and the PRAGUE-2 and DANAMI-2 studies collectively supported a safer profile of primary PCI as compared to thrombolysis by virtue of a reduced incidence of fatal stroke (haemorrhagic) and non-fatal re-infarction associated with the former strategy (Table 5.2). Differences in attitude as regards the use of PHF (and therefore of pharmacological reperfusion) can be recognized between the American and European guidelines also in their 2008 and 2007 updates of STEMI management: the ACC/AHA guidelines placed the emphasis on the speed and not the nature of reperfusion therapy that mainly improves the outcome of STEMI patients – accordingly no preference was expressed between pharmacological and mechanical reperfusion for the subgroup of early presenters – whilst the ESC sustained a more manifest inclination for an invasive reperfusion strategy. Of note, a paradox seems apparent between the European recommendations and the actual practice of PHF in Europe. A survey published in 2011 analysing data collected between 2003 and 2008 [16] shows that European countries such as UK, Sweden and France, have a wider usage of pharmacological reperfusion therapy initiated in the pre-hospital setting than regions in North America (Texas and Canada). Moreover, data from the Viennese and French registries, and a sub-group analysis of the CAPTIM conducted by a French group [52], all emphasized that a strategy of PHF is better than primary PCI in early-presenting patients, assuming that interventional facilities are available for possible rescue PCI (PCI performed in subjects with signs/symptoms of unsuccessful reperfusion) [17]. These evidence revealed that a pharmacological strategy for STEMI reperfusion has been largely adopted in Europe [17] despite the major emphasis on primary PCI expressed by the ESC in the 2003 STEMI guidelines and further reinforced in the latest versions. The recently published Strategic Reperfusion Early after Myocardial Infarction (STREAM) trial [53], whose results were not available at the time the contemporary guidelines were separately issued by the ACC/AHA and ESC Task Forces, further strengthen the value of PHF in patients presenting within 3 h after the onset of symptoms, by showing similar efficacy to primary PCI on a 30-day composite end-point of death from any cause, shock, congestive heart failure, or re-infarction (Table 5.2). How these data will impact on the next American and European guideline updates for STEMI management remains to be seen. Meanwhile, the STREAM study has re-opened the debate about whether primary PCI really is or is not superior to pre-hospital fibrinolysis, which has been improved in recent years by more widespread use of fibrin-specific agents as well as by more aggressive co-adjuvant anti-thrombotic therapy including DAPT (Table 5.2 reports the different medical regime adopted in the STREAM study compared with previous trials). Of note, the rates of re-infarction in the PHF and in the primary PCI arms were comparable in the STREAM population. The authors of the STREAM study cite the non-urgent nature of performing angiography in patients undergoing PHF as a factor giving rise to better reperfusion in these patients, since coronary bypass surgery was conducted more frequently than in subjects undergoing primary PCI, thus giving rise to more complete coronary revascularization. Moreover, all patients were admitted to catheterization-equipped hospitals, thus enabling immediate coronary intervention whenever indicated. In this way, the STREAM study re-launches the concept that fibrinolysis (particularly PHF) and PCI are not mutually exclusive as long as interventional procedures are conducted not in the immediate post-fibrinolysis period (within 1–2 h as part of a "facilitated" PCI strategy) and on a routine basis regardless of successful reperfusion by fibrinolytic therapy. It appears that early administration of fibrinolytic agents in the pre-hospital setting and subsequent transport of patients to a catheter laboratory-equipped facility (in a patient triage scheme that seems to resemble the one used in the early CAPTIM study [50]) may be of clinical utility in the management of STEMI patients, and certainly not of lesser efficacy than a primary PCI strategy [17].

TABLE 5.2 Comparison between fibrinolysis (with initiation in either the pre-hospital or in-hospital settings) and primary PCI on clinical outcomes

Trial	Study features	Thrombolytic agent	Co-adjuvant therapies	Death	Re-infarction	Bleedings/strokes
STREAM	N = 1,892 <3 h SO 30 days F/U	Tenecteplase (PHF)	Aspirin Clopidogrel Enoxaparin	500	334	500 (intracranial bleeding) (major bleeding)
CAPTIM	N = 840 <6 h SO 30 days F/U	Accelerated alteplase (PHF)	Aspirin (95.8 %) Heparin (97.4 %) Clopidogrel or Ticlopidine (59.8 %)	100 (All pts)	50 (All pts)	200 (hemorrhagic stroke) 67 (severe bleeding)
	(<2 hrs pts)			28.6 (<2 hrs pts)	−38.46 (< 2 hrs pts)	250 (severe hemorrhage) 80 (disabling stroke)
	(>2 hrs pts)			−45.45 (>2 hrs pts)	−83.3 (>2 hrs pts)	−26 (severe hemorrhage) 167 (disabling stroke)

(continued)

TABLE 5.2 (continued)

Trial	Study features	Thrombolytic agent	Co-adjuvant therapies	Death	Re-infarction	Bleedings/strokes
PRAGUE-2	N = 850 <12 h SO 30 days F/U	Streptokinase (in-hospital fibrinolysis)	Aspirin Fraxiparin Clopidogrel	1,000 (<3 hrs pts) 10.75 (3–12 hrs pts)	58.82 (All pts)	52.6 (non-fatal stroke) (All pts)
DANAMI-2	N = 1,572 <12 h SO 30 days F/U	Accelerated alteplase (in-hospital fibrinolysis)	Aspirin UFH I.v. Beta-blockers	–83.3	–21.3	111 (disabling stroke)

Data are reported as NNT (number needed to treat) to prevent death and re-infarction, and NNH (number needed to harm) for bleeding complications/strokes

F/U follow-up, *SO* symptom onset, *PHF* pre-hospital fibrinolysis, *UFH* unfractionated heparin, *<2 hrs pts*, *>2 hrs pts* patients presenting less than 2 or greater than 2 h after symptom onset

Timing of Reperfusion

Reperfusion therapy (either pharmacological or mechanical reperfusion) has to be initiated early in STEMI patients with onset of ischaemic symptoms within the previous 12 h – and the earlier within this time window that it is initiated, the better the outcome. In NSTEMI patients, only mechanical reperfusion is indicated, since fibrinolytic therapy appears to confer no benefit yet every possibility of harm, but the timing of intervention is still not well defined [1–4].

STEMI

In the early 2000s, the choice between PCI and fibrinolysis for STEMI was mainly determined by the facilities available at the patient's local hospital. Fibrinolytic therapy was the recommended reperfusion intervention in non-capable PCI hospitals, in order to avoid any potential delay in reperfusion time associated with transferring the patient to a catheterization laboratory. This approach has significantly changed over the years, due to an evolution in the definition of "timely reperfusion". In the 2004 ACC/AHA guidelines for STEMI [19], and in the following updates published in 2008 [20], the target medical contact–to-balloon or door-to-balloon interval was within 90 min, with the exception of patients presenting within 3 h from symptom onset, for whom PCI was indicated as first line option only if achieved within 60 min from FMC, otherwise immediate administration of thrombolytic therapy (within 30 min from FMC) was considered equally effective to a primary PCI approach. In the most recent version, the 2013 American guidelines [1] extended the time-window for medical contact–to-balloon up to 120 min, thus expanding the population of STEMI patients eligible for mechanical reperfusion therapy to those initially admitted to a PCI-incapable institution (Fig. 5.1). If patients are directly transported to a PCI-capable hospital, then the procedure has to be performed within 90 min. These figures are the same in the latest version of the European guidelines [2], and were already in the guidelines for myocardial revascularization issued by the ESC in 2008 [23]. Hence, a general consensus has developed over the years between Europe and North America in recognizing the superiority of primary PCI over fibrinolysis also in the early presenters (<3 h from symptom onset), and a view has emerged that PCI is less time-dependent than a medical reperfusion approach in restoring coronary patency. The Americans re-formulated their recommendation in the 2013 version of the STEMI guidelines based on data from the US National Registry of Myocardial Infarction (NRMI), which allowed a comparative analysis between onsite fibrinolysis in a PCI-incapable hospital and delayed PCI following transfer of patients to a catheterization facility [45]. These data demonstrated that transportation to a PCI-equipped institution achieved within 120 min offers advantages as regards mortality and re-infarction compared to onsite administration of fibrinolysis in a PCI-incapable centre. In the population of patients presenting within 2 h from symptom onset, the advantage of PCI over pharmacological reperfusion was also significant. Data analysis was conducted on a large and heterogeneous population of patients enrolled in the NRMI between 1994 and 2006. Over this period, the outcome from invasive procedures improved markedly, most likely attributable to advances in peri-procedural medical therapy, in particular the greater use of dual anti-platelet and anti-coagulant strategies.

NSTEMI/UA

In NSTEMI/UA, optimal timing for invasive procedures (diagnostic angiography and PCI) is less well defined. The 2008 ESC committee for myocardial revascularization [23] indicated 72 h as the time window within which to perform angiography in this group of patients, with the exception of high-risk patients (GRACE risk score >140) who should undergo urgent angiography within 24 h. Intervening with angiography (and PCI as appropriate) in NSTEMI/UA patients with a low-/moderate-risk score (GRACE <140) at earlier time points has failed to produce evidence of superiority compared to a delayed invasive approach, where conservative treatment is prioritised [54]. The major limiting factor in determining the optimal time for angiography in NSTEMI patients is related to the incidence of post-procedural MI [55] that negatively impacts on the overall benefit of an early invasive approach (mean 1.2 h) versus a delayed strategy (mean 21 h) [56]. Agreement is apparent between Americans and Europeans in their most recent guidelines, in that stabilization of patients and reduction in blood thrombogenicity achieved by intensive anti-platelet and anti-coagulant therapy in the acute phase has been advocated by both sets of guidelines in order to reduce the incidence of post-procedural ischaemic events. On the other hand, early intervention may prevent unstable plaques from progressing to the point of complete coronary occlusion. Hence, the timing for angiography +/− revascularization has to be tailored to individual cases, based on considerations of risk and hemodynamic stability. As a consequence, both sets of guidelines strongly advocate continuous monitoring of NSTEMI/UA patients for early signs of clinical complications that may require prompt intervention. The American guidelines for NSTEMI-UA specifically identify the criteria that qualify patients for early diagnostic angiography: recurrent symptoms/ischaemia, heart failure, or serious arrhythmias. For all other patients, stress testing is advocated to quantify risk; low-risk patients can be discharged with optimal preventative therapy, to undergo elective angiography, whilst those classified as high-risk should undergo early angiography. A similar approach can be recognized in the European guidelines. However, the ESC emphasize the importance of an early invasive approach to diabetic patients, who demonstrate a worse outcome that non-diabetic patients in many clinical trials [57], thus highlighting the need for aggressive and intensive medical therapy in this particular group for whom early revascularization should be considered. The ESC, but not the ACC/AHA Task Force, also express their preference for the use of the novel platelet inhibitors prasugrel and ticagrelor in diabetic patients in order to obtain a greater anti-platelet effect than that achieved with clopidogrel (as discussed below).

Of note, although the European and American guidelines differ slightly in their recommendations as to choice of reperfusion therapy (in STEMI) and the timing of intervention (in all ACS patients), a point of agreement that has emerged over the years is the notion that intensive anti-thrombotic medical management is required in all ACS patients as co-adjuvant therapy to improve clinical outcomes (Table 5.3).

Anti-thrombotic Therapy

Much of the clinical improvement achieved in the last decade in both prevention and treatment of ACS has to be attributed to advances in anti-thrombotic therapy, especially with development of new molecules with increased inhibitory effect on platelet activity. Figure 5.2 illustrates the targets of different anti-thrombotic drugs currently in use, comprising anti-platelet drugs (aspirin, $P2Y_{12}$-receptor antagonists and glycoprotein (Gp) IIb/IIIa inhibitors) and anti-coagulants (the direct thrombin inhibitor bivalirudin and indirect thrombin inhibitors namely heparins and fondaparinux).

Anti-platelets Drugs

Aspirin and $P2Y_{12}$-Receptor Inhibitors

Based on the Anti-Thrombotic Trialists Collaboration results [58], demonstrating the favourable effect of aspirin on incidence of vascular events in NSTEMI-ACS, and the ISIS-2 trial [39] reporting an additively favourable effect of aspirin and thrombolysis on outcome in STEMI patients, the 2003 European and 2004 American guidelines recommended administration of aspirin as first-line treatment in all ACS patients regardless of the strategy chosen (conservative or invasive). Anti-platelet therapy with aspirin has also demonstrated important benefits as regards mortality and progression to infarction in UA [59, 60]. The thienopyridine class of

TABLE 5.3 Anti-thrombotic therapies as co-adjuvants to medical and invasive treatments, and their place in long-term secondary prophylaxis, in STEMI and NSTEMI-ACS

	STEMI			NSTEMI	
	Acute phase PCI	TL	Long-term therapy	Acute phase	Long-term therapy
Aspirin	150–300 mg LD	150–300 mg LD	75 mg [ESC] 81 mg [ACC/AHA]	150–300 mg LD	75 mg [ESC] 81 mg [ACC/AHA]
P_2Y_{12} inhibitors: (one of the following)					
Clopidogrel	600 mg LD	300 mg LD	75 mg (12 months)	600 mg LD	75 mg (12 months)
Prasugrel	60 mg LD	Not indicated	10 mg (12 months)	Only if PCI planned 60 mg LD	Following PCI 10 mg (12 months)
Ticagrelor	180 mg LD	Not indicated	90 twice daily (12 months)	180 mg LD	90 twice daily (12 months)

(continued)

TABLE 5.3 (continued)

	STEMI			NSTEMI	
	Acute phase		Long-term therapy	Acute phase	Long-term therapy
	PCI	TL			
GpIIb/IIIa inhibitors (one of the following)					
Abciximab	Bolus of 0.25 mg/kg i.v. and 0.125 μg/kg/min infusion	Not indicated	Not indicated	Only if PCI planned Bolus of 0.25 mg/kg i.v. and 0.125 μg/kg/min infusion	Not indicated
Eptifibatide	Double bolus of 180 μg/kg i.v. and 2.0 μg/kg/min infusion			Double bolus of 180 μg/kg i.v. and 2.0 μg/kg/min infusion	
Tirofiban	25 μg/kg over 3 min i.v., followed by a maintenance infusion of 0.15 μg/kg/min			25 μg/kg over 3 min i.v., followed by a maintenance infusion of 0.15 μg/kg/min	

Heparins

LMWH (Enoxaparin)	0.5 mg/kg i.v. Bolus	30 mg i.v. Bolus+1 mg/kg twice daily subcutaneously	Not indicated (up to discharge)	1 mg/kg twice daily subcutaneously	Not indicated
UFH	i.v. bolus 60–70 IU/kg+infusion (aPTT 1.5–2.5 × control)	60 U/kg i.v. Bolus+infusion (aPTT 1.5–2.5 control)	Not indicated (up to 48 h)	i.v. bolus 60–70 IU/kg+infusion (aPTT 1.5–2.5 × control)	
Bivalirudin	0.75 mg/kg i.v. Bolu+1.75 mg/kg/h	No indicated	Not indicated (up to discharge)	ONLY if PCI planned 0.75 mg/kg i.v. Bolu+1.75 mg/kg/h	
Fondaparinux	Contraindicated	2.5 mg/daily subcutaneously	Not indicated (up to discharge)	2.5 mg/daily subcutaneously	

aPTT activated partial thromboplastin time, *LD* loading dose, *LMWH* low molecular weight heparin, *PCI* percutaneous coronary intervention, *TL* thrombolysis, *UFH* unfractionated heparin

FIGURE 5.2 Pharmacological targets of anti-thrombotic agents used in ACS. A thrombogenic surface (fibrinogen, von Willebrand Factor (*vWF*) and collagen) anchors platelets to the vascular wall by engaging specific platelet glycoproteins (Gps: GPIIb/IIIa, GpIb and GpVI respectively). The ensuing activation of platelets induced by integrin engagement, along with locally produced thrombin, leads to platelet activation and release of additional platelet-derived soluble thrombogenic molecules (ADP, thromboxane A_2 (TxA_2)) that are essential in stabilizing the initial aggregate, as they activate and recruit other circulating platelets and also produce a conformational change in GPIIb/IIIa from a low- to a high-affinity state for fibrinogen, which acts as a bridge between platelets. Activation of the coagulation cascade contributes to thrombus stabilization by promoting thrombin-mediated formation of fibrin cross-linking fibres. Aspirin reduces platelet TxA2 production through its inhibitory activity on cyclooxygenase-1. Thienopyridines and ticagrelor selectively bind the adenosine diphosphate (*ADP*) purinergic receptor $P2Y_{12}$ on platelets to permanently (thienopyridines) or reversibly (ticagrelor) inactivate it. GpIIb/IIIa inhibitors interfere with platelet-to-platelet interactions and platelet anchoring to the thrombogenic surface. Anti-coagulants mainly block thrombin activity either through a direct effect (bivalirudin) or via an indirect mechanism requiring anti-thrombin (*AT*) (heparins: low molecular weight heparin (*LMWH*) or unfractionated heparin (*UFH*)) or inhibiting Factor Xa required for its activation (fondaparinux). Note that thrombin also activates platelets through engagement of protease activated receptors (*PARs*). Co-administration of anti-platelets and anticoagulants interferes with platelet activation at multiple levels

anti-platelet agents (ticlopidine, a first generation drug, and subsequently clopidogrel, a second generation thienopyridine) was then developed, with the rationale of offering such drugs to patients with hypersensitivity or major gastrointestinal intolerance to aspirin; these drugs (or more precisely, their active metabolites) irreversibly bind and block the ADP platelet receptor $P2Y_{12}$. Hence, the 2003 ESC and 2004 ACC/AHA guidelines also advocate the use of ticlopidine or clopidogrel as co-adjuvant anti-platelet agents with thrombolysis in patients with allergy to aspirin, but no specific

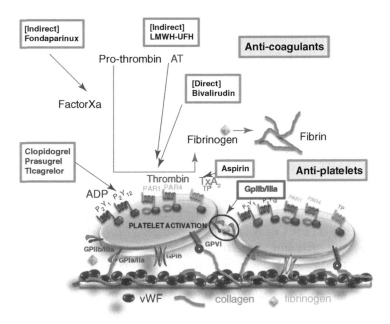

recommendations were given for the use of ADP antagonists in primary PCI (either as co-adjuvant therapy or in the post-procedural phase) due to lack of clinical evidence at that time. Ancillary therapy to primary PCI consisted of anti-coagulant drugs (mainly heparins) and Gp IIb/IIIa antagonists (as expanded upon below). The add-on value of aspirin to fibrinolysis was reinforced by the CLARITY-TIMI 28 study published in 2005 [61]. Therefore, the subsequent updates in 2007 of STEMI management issued by the ESC and ACC/AHA Task Forces further underlined the important role of anti-platelet therapy with aspirin in conjunction with fibrinolytic reperfusion therapy on the main clinical outcomes of mortality and re-infarction in STEMI patients. At the same time, advances in the understanding of platelet activation, and the notion that inhibition of platelet activity at multiple levels could offer additive or even synergistic anti-platelet effect, prompted investigators to address the potential advantage of thienopyridine-aspirin co-administration on clinical outcomes in ACS. Two major trials, CLARITY-TIMI 28 [61] and COMMIT-CCS-2 [34], provided clear evidence for a net benefit of clopidogrel (which by that time had supplanted ticlopidine in clinical use due to a high incidence of haematological toxicities with ticlopidine) as add-on therapy to aspirin, in patients treated with either fibrinolysis or PCI. This benefit was mainly related to reduction of re-infarction rates. The COMMIT trial also showed superiority of DAPT versus aspirin alone in ACS patients not undergoing reperfusion therapy, whether pharmacological or invasive. These data prompted the introduction in the 2008 ACC/AHA and 2007 ESC updates of DAPT for all ACS patients, be they STEMI or NSTEMI, regardless of reperfusion strategy and including those treated by a conservative approach. The recommended length of treatment was restricted to the short-term follow-up length of these two trials (30 days), although the possibility was advanced that substantial benefit may accrue from DAPT in longer-term therapy. The evidence that benefit is indeed obtained by continuing DAPT for at least 12 months post-acute event increased in the following years (Table 5.4), and it is now stated in the most recent American and European guidelines that DAPT should continue for 12 months after presentation with ACS (whilst the beneficial effect of DAPT is not greater if continued for longer than 1 year, at least in patients receiving drug-eluting stents [73]). Exceptions are for patients with ischaemic stroke and transient ischaemic attack, for whom DAPT is contraindicated/not recommended because of increased bleeding events.

Major issues have since arisen with regard to inter-individual variability of platelet response to clopidogrel, as a consequence of variations in liver metabolism that is required to convert the pro-drug to the active molecule. Co-administration of other drugs metabolized by hepatic cytochrome P450 (CYP), chiefly statins and proton-pump inhibitors [74–77], and genetic variants of CYP-2C19 [78–80], have been reported in a number of studies to be associated

TABLE 5.4 Summary of trials showing the effect of P2Y$_{12}$-receptor antagonists (alone or in DAPT) on clinical outcomes

Trial	Study population	Treatment	Follow-up	End-point	NNT	NNH
Long-term outcomes [STEMI/NSTEMI]						
CURE [62]	12,562 pts with NSTEMI	Clopidogrel + aspirin vs Placebo + aspirin (Aspirin dose 75–325 mg)	12 months	CV death, MI, or stroke	53	91
					333	167
					26	83
CREDO [63]	2,116 pts scheduled for elective PCI	Clopidogrel vs placebo Aspirin in all pts (81–325 mg)	12 months	CV death, MI, or stroke	33	48
PCI-CURE [64]	2,658 pts with NSTEMI undergoing PCI	Clopidogrel vs placebo (aspirin in all pts (75–325 mg)	12 months	CV death, MI, or Stroke	31	–250
					–143	–
					53	83
TRITON-TIMI 38 [65]	13,608 pts with ACS scheduled for PCI	Prasugrel (60 LD + 10 mg) vs clopidogrel (300 LD + 75 mg) Aspirin in all pts (75–162 mg)	15 months	CV death, MI, or stroke	45	45

(continued)

TABLE 5.4 (continued)

Trial	Study population	Treatment	Follow-up	End-point	NNT	NNH
PLATO [66]	18,624 pts with STEMI (38 %) AND NSTEMI (59 %) for early PCI	Ticagrelor (180 LD+90 mg bid) vsclopidogrel (300–600 LD+75 mg) Aspirin in all pts (75–162 mg)	12 months	Death, MI, or stroke	52.6	−250
PLATO-PCI [67]	13,408 pts with STEMI (49.1 %) and NSTEMI (50.99 %)	Ticagrelor (180 LD+90 mg bid) vs clopidogrel (300–600 LD+75 mg) Aspirin in all pts (75–162 mg)	12 months	Death, MI, or stroke	58.5	1,000
Short-term outcomes [STEMI/NSTEMI]						
CLARITY [61]	3,491 pts with STEMI	Clopidogrel+aspirin vs Placebo+aspirin (Aspirin dose 150–325 mg)	30 days	Death, recurrent MI	16	500
COMMIT [34]	45,852 pts with MI	Clopidogrel+aspirin vs Placebo+aspirin (Aspirin dose 162 mg)	15 days	Death Re-infarction Stroke	11	333
PCI-CLARITY [68]	1,863 pts with STEMI undergoing PCI	Clopidogrel+aspirin vs Placebo+aspirin (Aspirin dose 150–325 mg)	30 days	Death, recurrent MI, or stroke	22	100

Study	Population	Comparison	Follow-up	Endpoint	NNT	NNH
CURRENT/OASIS [69]	25,086 pts with STEMI/NSTEMI undergoing early PCI (within 72 h)	Clopidogrel double dose (600 mg LD+150 maintenance) vs Clopidogrel standard dose (300 mg LD+75 mg)	30 days	CV death, MI, or stroke	30	20.53
Secondary long-term prevention in high risk PTS						
MATCH [70]	7,599 high-risk pts	Aspirin vs placebo Clopidogrel in all pts (75 mg)	18 months	Ischaemic stroke, MI, vascular death, rehospitalisation	100	77
CHARISMA [71]	15,603 pts with multiple risk factors or evident CV disease	Clopidogrel vs placebo Aspirin in all pts (75–162 mg)	28 months	CV death, MI, or stroke	200	250
CAPRIE [72]	19,185 pts with previous CV events and/or manifest atherosclerotic disease	Clopidogrel vs aspirin	1.91 year	CV death, MI, or stroke	111	–10,000

CV cardiovascular, *MI* myocardial infarction, *LD* loading dose, *PCI* percutaneous coronary intervention, *NNT* number needed-to-treat, *NNH* number needed-to-harm with reduced biotransformation of clopidogrel to its active metabolite – and, at least in the case of the genetic slow-metabolizer variants of CYP-2C19, have been demonstrated to give rise to impaired platelet inhibitory effects in response to clopidogrel. Therefore the third generation thienopyridine prasugrel was developed, which is less dependent on hepatic metabolism since it requires a single pass liver conversion into its active metabolite compared with the two-step hepatic bio-transformation of clopidopgrel [17, 18]. In an attempt to clarify the important aspects of pharmacogenetics and drug interactions of thienopyridines, the ACCF/ACG/AHA societies recently reviewed the evidence-base in the literature on the use of thienopyridines in ACS in 2010 [81]. The consensus document summarizes three main aspects of importance to medical practitioners: (1) DAPT increases the risk of gastro-intestinal bleeds compared to aspirin monotherapy; (2) it is possible and advisable to prevent the increased risk of gastro-intestinal bleeding complications in patients receiving DAPT by concomitant administration of a proton-pump inhibitor (since, although proton pump inhibitors do impair clopidogrel biotransformation, this does not appear to translate to a clini-cally important effect as demonstrated in recent large clinical trials [82, 83]; (3) the relationship between genetic variations in CYP and reduced bioconversion of clopidogrel is clear, but whether this phenomenon has meaningful clinical conse-quences remains uncertain. Overall the statement endorses the use of proton pump inhibitors in combination with clopi-dogrel, in light of a net benefit deriving from prevention of gastrointestinal bleeding in patients on DAPT which is not counterbalanced by a demonstrated negative impact on clini-cal outcomes. In agreement with this, the 2012 American guidelines for STEMI and the 2011 updates for NSTEMI/UA further reinforce the need to consider proton pump inhibitor co-administration with DAPT in patients at risk of gastro-intestinal bleeding, as this increases drug tolerability and adher-ence to therapy by patients, with consequent favourable effects on the prevention of re-infarction or re-stenosis fol-lowing ACS. The ESC guidelines agree in this respect.

More recently, in order to bypass the liver metabolism-dependent activation step that can delay the onset of action of thienopyridines, and in order to achieve reversible antagonism of ADP which may be useful in patients on DAPT requiring surgical intervention or experiencing bleeding, ticagrelor was launched [18]. This drug, a cyclopentyltriazolopyrimidine (therefore chemically different from the thienopyridines), is a reversible $P2Y_{12}$ antagonist which does not require biotransformation for its activity.

The latest versions of the American and European guidelines both mention prasugrel and ticagrelor in the context of STEMI and NSTEMI/UA management. However, discrepancies over which $P2Y_{12}$ antagonist to use in different clinical settings can be recognized between the American and European recommendations. The ESC guidelines promote the use of prasugrel and ticagrelor instead of clopidogrel as part of DAPT co-adjuvant to PCI, based on the favourable effect of prasugrel and ticagrelor compared with clopidogrel on primary outcomes demonstrated in the TRITON TIMI-38 and PLATO trials respectively [65–67]. Diabetic patients are singled out as those who may mainly benefit from the use of these more efficacious anti-platelet drugs. The ACC/AHA Task Force have exhibited a more cautious attitude in replacing clopidogrel with prasugrel or ticagrelor, in view of more bleeding events associated with the newer drugs compared with clopidogrel (Table 5.4) that may negatively impact on any benefit accrued. In years to come, more clinical evidence will become available on the benefits and risks of these different anti-platelet regimes, allowing their risk/benefit ratio to be better elucidated in long-term follow-up. Of note, the TRITON TIMI-38 study compared prasugrel to clopidogrel used at a loading dose that is below that currently recommended (600 mg) for PCI. Moreover, at present no data are available as regards the use of the new $P2Y_{12}$ antagonists in the setting of fibrinolysis, for which both the ESC and ACC/AHA Task Forces maintain the previous recommendation of aspirin in combination with clopidogrel as DAPT (Table 5.3).

GpIIb/IIIa Inhibitors

There is agreement between the European and American guidelines that, with the now widespread use of DAPT, and the recent availability of ever more potent anti-platelet drugs, the value of GpIIb/IIIa inhibitors in ACS is much less than previously. Abciximab has been the most widely used GpIIa/IIIa inhibitor in the setting of ACS. When tested as a co-adjuvant to fibrinolysis with streptokinase in two early randomized clinical trials, it failed to demonstrate additive benefit on 30-day mortality, although a slight reduction in re-infarction during in-hospital stay was seen albeit at the price of increased bleeding complications [84, 85]. Based on such evidence, the 2003 ESC Task Force did not promote the routine use of GpIIb/IIIa inhibitors as ancillary therapy to fibrinolysis in STEMI and no change has arisen in later updates. In the setting of primary PCI, conflicting data have been published as regards the favourable effect of GpIIa/IIIa inhibitors on top of aspirin and anti-coagulants, prior to the routine use of DAPT [86, 87]. Moreover, in the recent BRAVE-3 trial [88], that tested the usefulness of GpIIb/IIIa inhibition with abciximab added on to clopidogrel 600 mg (with co-administration of aspirin and heparin) in STEMI patients undergoing PCI, abciximab failed to reduce infarct size compared with optimal DAPT. On the other hand, no harmful effect of GpIIb/IIIa inhibition was seen in terms of bleeding complications in this study. Hence, in the most recent guidelines issued by ESC and ACC/AHA, GpIIb/IIIa inhibition is referred to simply as a reasonable choice for STEMI/NSTEMI patients undergoing invasive procedures, and no specific preference is expressed for abciximab or the other GpIIb/IIIa inhibitors currently available (tirofiban and eptifibatide).

Anti-coagulant Drugs

Unlike anti-platelet drugs, which are indicated not only in the acute phase but also in the long-term treatment of ACS, anti-coagulation is indicated in the acute phase only. In the 2004

American STEMI guidelines the choice was between heparins (unfractionated and low molecular weight heparins) and bivalirudin. They were termed anti-thrombins because of their mechanism of action, that consists of blockade of the enzymatic activity of thrombin (i.e. conversion of soluble fibrinogen to insoluble fibrin), either through direct binding of the drug to the active domain of thrombin (for bivalirudin) or through an indirect action that requires anti-thrombin (AT) as a co-factor to inhibit the enzymatic activity of thrombin (for heparins) [89]. However, the nomenclature was reviewed in the subsequent 2007 update of the STEMI guidelines in recognition of the ability of the heparins to bind a number of plasma proteins other than thrombin that contribute to the coagulation cascade [90], and the term anti-thrombins was replaced by anti-coagulants.

Anti-coagulants are recommended in all ACS patients, regardless of STEMI or NSTEMI diagnosis, and regardless of the management strategy selected (invasive or non–invasive). In the 2004 American STEMI consensus document, heparins were preferred to bivalirudin, this latter indicated as an alternative option in patients with known heparin-induced thrombocytopenia. The low molecular weight heparin enoxaparin was seen to offer advantages over unfractionated heparin, especially when the duration of anti-coagulation was longer than 48 h. For primary PCI, unfractionated heparin was the recommended choice, since no clinical trials specifically addressing the impact of low molecular weight heparin on outcomes in this setting were available. As an adjuvant to fibrinolysis, the role of anti-coagulants was more controversial, and they were specifically recommended as co-adjuvant to fibrin-specific lytic agents, since no clear additive benefit was found for heparins in co-administration with streptokinase [84]. Bivalirudin was not approved at that time for use in Europe. Therefore, the 2003 ESC guidelines advocated only heparins as anti-coagulants, emphasizing their clinical utility in STEMI patients undergoing fibrinolytic reperfusion, with no clear preference between unfractionated and low molecular weight heparin. For primary PCI, no recommendation for heparin treatment was given. Over the ensuing years, accumulating evidence has supported the additive benefit of anti-coagulants to both fibrinolytics and PCI. The EXTRACT-TIMI 23 study [91] reinforced the data previously published in the ASSENT-3 trial [84], showing that enoxaparin is superior to unfractionated heparin in patients treated with fibrin-specific lytic agents but not in streptokinase treated patients.

A newly developed anti-coagulant fondaparinux, that selectively binds anti-thrombin III to induce a conformational change resulting in enhanced inhibitory activity on factor Xa, was tested in the OASIS-6 study [92]. The results, published in 2006, demonstrated similar efficacy of fondaparinux and enoxaparin on the primary end-points (death, MI and stroke at 9, 30 days and 6 months) in patients undergoing either pharmacological or mechanical reperfusion therapy, or neither. As a consequence, fondaparinux was recommended as an alternative anti-coagulant in both the 2007 ACC/AHA and 2008 ESC guidelines for STEMI, although caution was expressed because of an increased risk of catheter thrombosis related to fondaparinux use that emerged in the OASIS-6 study , leading the writing committees to discourage its use as sole anti-coagulant in patients undergoing mechanical reperfusion (suggesting co-treatment with a GpIIb/IIIa inhibitor instead). The most recent versions of the STEMI guidelines in Europe and North America both reinforce the harmful effect of fondaparinux in primary PCI, and advise administration of unfractionated heparin before invasive procedures are carried out in patients who previously received fondaparinux only.

Unlike the consensus expressed for fondaparinux, the ESC and ACC/AHA guidelines differ in their preference for other anti-coagulants in the context of primary PCI. The American guidelines underline the failure of enoxaparin to show a superior effect over unfractionated heparin on primary end-points in the ATOLL trial [93], whilst the European guidelines emphasize that, although no differences were observed between the two anti-coagulant regimes in this trial (in terms of mortality at 30 days, complications of MI, procedural failure or major bleeding), the secondary end-point (composite of death, recurrent ACS and urgent revascularization) showed superiority for the enoxaparin arm. Also for bivalirudin the views differ. Although bivalirudin produced less bleeding complications than unfractionated heparin in the HORIZON-AMI trial [94], this was at the price of increased rates of stent thrombosis, and this latter aspect is emphasized by the American guidelines which therefore express caution in the use of bivalirudin in place of heparins in primary PCI. The European guidelines emphasize their view that increased restenosis can be overcome by more potent DAPT, since in the HORIZON-AMI trial bivalirudin was administered in conjunction with a loading dose of clopidogrel at 300 mg rather than 600 mg. Moreover, given the reduction in bleeding complications with bivalirudin, the European guidelines suggest it as a valid alternative in patients for whom GpIIb/IIIa inhibition is to be avoided (due to increased risk of bleeding).

Agreement is expressed on the need to use anti-coagulant therapy for peri-procedural prophylaxis of thrombo-embolic events (including deep venous thrombosis, pulmonary embolism, left ventricular mural thrombus formation and cerebral embolism). No requirement is propounded for prolonged administration of anti-coagulants post-PCI. Similarly, in NSTEMI/UA patients who do not undergo invasive therapy, anti-coagulants are advocated for the duration of their hospital stay, up to 8 days (or in the case of unfractionated heparin for 48 h maximum), given the limited benefit of anti-coagulation as regards long-term clinical outcomes with a considerable increase in bleeding complications [95].

Long-Term Therapy

The long-term management of ACS relies on preventative measures (both pharmacological and non-pharmacological) to reduce the occurrence of future thrombotic events. Correction of classical cardiovascular risk factors with life-style modifications (including a cardiac rehabilitation programme where appropriate), anti-hypertensive and lipid-lowering therapies are all crucial components following STEMI or NSTEMI/UA, and these measures all help to reduce blood thrombogenicity. Indeed, evidence exists that all cardiovascular risk factors increase platelet activity as well as inflammation [96, 97], thus predisposing to both athero-sclerosis progression and superadded thrombosis. Additionally, as mentioned above, anti-platelet drugs are an important aspect of the long-term management of these patients, and the need for more intensive platelet inhibition in secondary prevention than that achieved with aspirin monotherapy has been particularly emphasized in the most recent guidelines; DAPT is now recommended in the long-term therapy of ACS up to 1 year, and not just as a reasonable choice as reported in previous versions [1–4].

Compared with previous versions, the most recent recommendations do not differ in optimal blood pressure and serum cholesterol targets (blood pressure <140/90 mmHg and <130/80 mmHg in diabetics; low-density lipoprotein cholesterol <70 mg/dl (<1.75 mmol/L)). Unlike the American guidelines, the ESC Task Force specifically addresses long-term prophylaxis in selected groups of patients who are considered at particularly high cardiovascular risk and who therefore merit particular attention, namely diabetics and patients with impaired renal function (glomerular filtration rate <60 ml/min). These groups of patients are identified as those for whom prasugrel (in diabetics) and ticagrelor (in patients with impaired renal function) may offer particular advantages over clopidogrel, on the basis of the results from the TRITON TIMI-38 and PLATO studies [65–67]. As mentioned above, the American guidelines express no preference for any $P2Y_{12}$ receptor antagonist over any other, in DAPT.

Conclusion

The development of novel anti-thrombotic drugs has contributed significantly to the evolution of management approaches to ACS over the last decade. The modern management of

STEMI and NSTEMI/UA patients is based on a combined pharmacological approach using multiple drugs with different therapeutic targets, either alone or in combination with an invasive strategy. This approach has led to important benefits on mortality and morbidity rates associated with ACS, both in the acute and long-term phases. Nevertheless, the benefits of intensive anti-thrombotic (comprising both anti-platelet and anti-coagulant) therapy is counterbalanced to some degree by increased risk of bleeding complications, that needs to be taken into account when tailoring therapy to the individual patient. The American and European guidelines are important sources of evidence-based clinical recommendations, and the succession of updates issued over the last decade reflect both the exponential rise in information derived from clinical research and from progress in available medical and interventional therapies achieved over the years. In their latest versions, a very similar approach to the treatment of ACS can be seen in both the European and American guidelines. However, subtle discrepancies are present and relate to differences in data interpretation, especially where the available evidence comes from single trials only (e.g. PLATO for ticagrelor, TRITON TIMI-38 for prasugrel). The fact that such discrepancies in their points of view exist is a clear indication that additional data are required in order to elucidate more robustly the true benefits versus risks of emerging treatment approaches in these patients.

References

1. O'Gara PT, Kushner FG, Ascheim DD, et al. 2013 ACCF/AHA Guideline for the Management of ST-Elevation Myocardial Infarction: A Report of the American College of Cardiology Foundation/American Heart Association Task Force on Practice Guidelines. Circulation. 2013;127:e362–425.
2. Steg PG, James SK, Atar D, et al. ESC Guidelines for the management of acute myocardial infarction in patients presenting with ST-segment elevation. Task Force on the management of ST-segment elevation acute myocardial infarction of the European Society of Cardiology (ESC). Eur Heart J. 2012;33:2569–619.

3. Jneid H, Anderson JL, Wright RS, et al. 2012 ACCF/AHA focused update of the guideline for the management of patients with unstable angina/non -ST-elevation myocardial infarction (updating the 2007 guideline and replacing the 2011 focused update): a report of the American College of Cardiology Foundation/American Heart Association Task Force on practice guidelines. Circulation. 2012;126:875–910.

4. Hamm CW, Bassand JP, Agewall S, et al. ESC guidelines for the management of acute coronary syndromes in patients presenting without persistent ST-segment elevation: the task force for the management of acute coronary syndromes (ACS) in patients presenting without persistent ST-segment elevation of the European Society of Cardiology. ESC Eur Heart J. 2011;32(23):2999–3054.

5. Ryan TJ, Anderson JL, Antman EM, et al. ACC/AHA guidelines for the management of patients with acute myocardial infarction. A report of the American College of Cardiology/American Heart Association Task Force on practice guidelines (committee on management of acute myocardial infarction). J Am Coll Cardiol. 1996;28(5):1328–428.

6. Acute myocardial infarction: pre-hospital and in-hospital management. The Task Force on the Management of Acute Myocardial Infarction of the European Society of Cardiology. Eur Heart J. 1996;17(1):43–63.

7. Braunwald E, Antman EM, Beasley JW, et al. ACC/AHA guidelines for the management of patients with unstable angina and non-ST-segment elevation myocardial infarction: executive summary and recommendations. A report of the American College of Cardiology/American Heart Association Task Force on practice guidelines (committee on the management of patients with unstable angina). Circulation. 2000;102(10):1193–209.

8. Van de Werf F, Ardissino D, Betriu A, et al. Management of acute myocardial infarction in patients presenting with ST-segment elevation. The task force on the management of acute myocardial infarction of the European Society of Cardiology. Eur Heart J. 2003;24(1):28–66.

9. The Joint European Society of Cardiology/American College of Cardiology Committee. Myocardial infarction redefined—a consensus document of the Joint European Society of Cardiology/American College of Cardiology Committee for the redefinition of myocardial infarction. Eur Heart J. 2000;21:1502–13.

10. Thygesen K, Alpert JS, White HD, et al. Universal definition of myocardial infarction. Joint ESC/ACCF/AHA/WHF task force for the redefinition of myocardial infarction. Eur Heart J. 2007;28(20):2525–38.

11. Thygesen K, Alpert JS, Jaffe AS, et al. Third universal definition of myocardial infarction. Circulation. 2012;126(16):2020–35.

12. Levine GN, Bates ER, Blankenship JC, et al. 2011 ACCF/AHA/ SCAI guideline for percutaneous coronary intervention: a report of the American College of Cardiology Foundation/American Heart Association Task Force on practice guidelines and the society for cardiovascular angiography and interventions. Circulation. 2011;124(23):e574–651.

13. Wijns W, Kolh P, Danchin N, et al. Guidelines on myocardial revascularization. Task force on myocardial revascularization of the European Society of Cardiology (ESC) and the European association for cardio-thoracic surgery (EACTS); European association for percutaneous cardiovascular interventions (EAPCI). Eur Heart J. 2010;31(20):2501–55.

14. Andersen HR, Nielsen TT, Rasmussen K, et al. A comparison of coronary angioplasty with fibrinolytic therapy in acute myocardial infarction. N Engl J Med. 2003;349(8):733–42.

15. Busk M, Maeng M, Rasmussen K, Kelbaek H, et al. The Danish multicentre randomized study of fibrinolytic therapy vs. primary angioplasty in acute myocardial infarction (the DANAMI-2 trial): outcome after 3 years follow-up. Eur Heart J. 2008;29(10):1259–66.

16. Huynh T, Birkhead J, Huber K, et al. The pre-hospital fibrinolysis experience in Europe and North America and implications for wider dissemination. JACC Cardiovasc Interv. 2011;4(8):877–83.

17. Passacquale G, Ferro A. Oral antiplatelet agents clopidogrel and prasugrel for the prevention of cardiovascular events. BMJ. 2011;342:d3488.

18. Floyd CN, Passacquale G, Ferro A. Comparative pharmacokinetics and pharmacodynamics of platelet adenosine diphosphate receptor antagonists and their clinical implications. Clin Pharmacokinet. 2012;51(7):429–42.

19. Van de Werf F, Bax J, Betriu A, et al. Management of acute myocardial infarction in patients presenting with persistent ST-segment elevation: the task force on the management of ST-segment elevation acute myocardial infarction of the European Society of Cardiology. Eur Heart J. 2008;29:2909–45.

20. Antman EM, Hand M, Armstrong PW, et al. 2007 Focused update of the ACC/AHA 2004 guidelines for the management of patients with ST-elevation myocardial infarction: a report of the American College of Cardiology/American Heart Association Task Force on practice guidelines: developed in collaboration with the Canadian cardiovascular society endorsed by the American academy of family physicians: 2007 writing group to review new evidence and update the ACC/AHA 2004 guidelines for the management of patients with ST-elevation myocardial infarction, writing on behalf of the 2004 writing committee. Circulation. 2008;117(2):296–329.

21. Meine TJ, Roe MT, Chen AY, et al. Association of intravenous morphine use and outcomes in acute coronary syndromes: results from

the CRUSADE Quality Improvement Initiative. Am Heart J. 2005;149(6):1043–9.

22. Gross GJ, Gross ER, Peart JN. Association of intravenous morphine use and outcomes in acute coronary syndromes: results from the CRUSADE Quality Improvement Initiative. Am Heart J. 2005;150(6):e3.

23. Antman EM, Anbe DT, Armstrong PW, et al. ACC/AHA guidelines for the management of patients with ST-elevation myocardial infarction–executive summary. A report of the American College of Cardiology/American Heart Association Task Force on Practice Guidelines (Writing Committee to revise the 1999 guidelines for the management of patients with acute myocardial infarction). J Am Coll Cardiol. 2004;44(3):671–719.

24. Gislason GH, Jacobsen S, Rasmussen JN, et al. Risk of death or reinfarction associated with the use of selective cyclooxygenase-2 inhibitors and nonselective nonsteroidal antiinflammatory drugs after acute myocardial infarction. Circulation. 2006;113:2906–13.

25. McGettigan P, Henry D. Cardiovascular risk and inhibition of cyclo-oxygenase: a systematic review of the observational studies of selective and nonselective inhibitors of cyclooxygenase 2. JAMA. 2006;296:1633–44.

26. Kearney PM, Baigent C, Godwin J, et al. Do selective cyclo-oxygen-ase-2 inhibitors and traditional non-steroidal anti-inflammatory drugs increase the risk of atherothrombosis? Meta-analysis of randomised trials. BMJ. 2006;332:1302–8.

27. Antman EM, Bennett JS, Daugherty A, et al. Use of nonsteroidal antiinflammatory drugs: an update for clinicians: a scientific statement from the American Heart Association. Circulation. 2007;115:1634–42.

28. Randomised trial of intravenous atenolol among 16,027 cases of suspected acute myocardial infarction: ISIS-1. First International Study of Infarct Survival Collaborative Group. Lancet. 1986;2:57–66.

29. The MIAMI Trial Research Group. Metoprolol in acute myocardial infarction: patient population. Am J Cardiol. 1985;56:10G–4.

30. The TIMI Study Group. Comparison of invasive and conservative strategies after treatment with intravenous tissue plasminogen activator in acute myocardial infarction: results of the thrombolysis in myocardial infarction (TIMI) phase II trial. N Engl J Med. 1989;320:618–27.

31. Roberts R, Rogers WJ, Mueller HS, et al. Immediate versus deferred beta-blockade following thrombolytic therapy in patients with acute myocardial infarction: results of the Thrombolysis in Myocardial Infarction (TIMI) II-B Study. Circulation. 1991;83:422–37.

32. Van de Werf F, Janssens L, Brzostek T, et al. Short-term effects of early intravenous treatment with a beta-adrenergic blocking agent

or a specific bradycardiac agent in patients with acute myocardial infarction receiving thrombolytic therapy. J Am Coll Cardiol. 1993;22:407–16.

33. Pfisterer M, Cox JL, Granger CB, et al. Atenolol use and clinical outcomes after thrombolysis for acute myocardial infarction: the GUSTO-I experience. Global Utilization of Streptokinase and TPA (alteplase) for Occluded Coronary Arteries. J Am Coll Cardiol. 1998;32:634–40.

34. Chen ZM, Pan HC, Chen YP, et al. Early intravenous then oral metoprolol in 45,852 patients with acute myocardial infarction: randomized placebo-controlled trial. Lancet. 2005;366:1622–32.

35. Brandler E, Paladino L, Sinert R. Does the early administration of beta-blockers improve the in-hospital mortality rate of patients admitted with acute coronary syndrome? Acad Emerg Med. 2010;17:1–10.

36. GISSI-3: effects of lisinopril and transdermal glyceryl trinitrate singly and together on 6-week mortality and ventricular function after acute myocardial infarction. Gruppo Italiano per lo Studio della Sopravvivenza nell'infarto Miocardico. Lancet. 1994;343(8906):1115–22.

37. ISIS-4: a randomised factorial trial assessing early oral captopril, oral mononitrate, and intravenous magnesium sulphate in 58,050 patients with suspected acute myocardial infarction. ISIS-4 (Fourth International Study of Infarct Survival) Collaborative Group. Lancet. 1995;345(8951):669–85.

38. The European Myocardial Infarction Project Group. Prehospital thrombolytic therapy in patients with suspected acute myocardial infarction. N Engl J Med. 1993;329:383–9.

39. ISIS-2 (Second International Study of Infarct Survival) Collaborative Group. Randomised trial of intravenous streptokinase, oral aspirin, both or neither among 17,187 cases of suspected acute myocardial infarction: ISIS-2. Lancet. 1998;2:349–60.

40. TIMI IIIB Investigators. Effects of tissue plasminogen activator and comparison of early invasive and conservative strategies in unstable angina and non-Q wave myocardial infarction. Results of the TIMI IIIB Trial. Circulation. 1994;89:1545.

41. White HD, Van de Werf FJ. Thrombolysis for acute myocardial infarction. Circulation. 1998;97:1632–46.

42. Morrison LJ, Verbeek PR, McDonald AC, et al. Mortality and prehospital thrombolysis for acute myocardial infarction: a meta-analysis. JAMA. 2000;283(20):2686–92.

43. Assessment of the Safety and Efficacy of a New Thrombolytic (ASSENT-2) Investigators. Single-bolus tenecteplase compared with front-loaded alteplase in acute myocardial infarction: the ASSENT-2 double-blind randomised trial. Lancet. 1999;354:716–22.

44. Wallentin L, Goldstein P, Armstrong PW, et al. Efficacy and safety of tenecteplase in combination with the low-molecular-weight heparin enoxaparin or unfractionated heparin in the prehospital setting: the Assessment of the Safety and Efficacy of a New Thrombolytic Regimen (ASSENT)-3 PLUS randomized trial in acute myocardial infarction. Circulation. 2003;108(2):135–42.

45. Pinto DS, Frederick PD, Chakrabarti AK, et al. Benefit of transferring ST-segment-elevation myocardial infarction patients for percutaneous coronary intervention compared with administration of onsite fibrinolytic declines as delays increase. Circulation. 2011;124:2512–21.

46. The GUSTO Investigators. An international randomized trial comparing four thrombolytic strategies for acute myocardial infarction. N Engl J Med. 1993;329:673–82.

47. The Global Use of Strategies to Open Occluded Coronary Arteries (GUSTO III) Investigators. A comparison of reteplase with alteplase for acute myocardial infarction. N Engl J Med. 1997;337:1118–23.

48. Steg PG, Laperche T, Golmard JL, et al. Efficacy of streptokinase, but not tissue-type plasminogen activator, in achieving 90-minute patency after thrombolysis for acute myocardial infarction decreases with time to treatment. PERM Study Group. Prospective Evaluation of Reperfusion Markers. J Am Coll Cardiol. 1998;31(4):776–9.

49. Assessment of the Safety and Efficacy of a New Treatment Strategy with Percutaneous Coronary Intervention (ASSENT-4 PCI) investigators. Primary versus tenecteplase-facilitated percutaneous coronary intervention in patients with ST-segment elevation acute myocardial infarction (ASSENT-4 PCI): randomised trial. Lancet. 2006;367(9510):569–78.

50. Bonnefoy E, Lapostolle F, Leizorovicz A, et al. Primary angioplasty versus prehospital fibrinolysis in acute myocardial infarction: a randomised study. Lancet. 2002;360(9336):825–9.

51. Widimský P, Budesinský T, Vorác D, et al. Long distance transport for primary angioplasty vs immediate thrombolysis in acute myocardial infarction: final results of the randomized national multicentre trial-PRAGUE-2. Eur Heart J. 2003;24:94–104.

52. Steg PG, Bonnefoy E, Chabaud S, et al. Impact of time to treatment on mortality after prehospital fibrinolysis or primary angioplasty: data from the CAPTIM randomized clinical trial. Circulation. 2003;108(23):2851–6.

53. Armstrong PW, Gershlick AH, Goldstein P, et al. Fibrinolysis or primary PCI in ST-segment elevation myocardial infarction. N Engl J Med. 2013;368(15):1379–87.

54. Mehta SR, Granger CB, Boden WE, et al. Early versus delayed invasive intervention in acute coronary syndromes. N Engl J Med. 2009;360(21):2165–75.

55. Riezebos RK, Ronner E, Ter Bals E, et al. Immediate versus deferred coronary angioplasty in non-ST-segment elevation acute coronary syndromes. Heart. 2009;95:807–12.
56. Montalescot G, Cayla G, Collet JP, et al. Immediate vs delayed intervention for acute coronary syndromes: a randomized clinical trial. JAMA. 2009;302:947–54.
57. Dotevall A, Hasdai D, Wallentin L, Battler A, Rosengren A. Diabetes mellitus: clinical presentation and outcome in men and women with acute coronary syndromes. Data from the Euro Heart Survey ACS. Diabet Med. 2005;22:1542–50.
58. Antithrombotic Trialists' Collaboration. Collaborative metaanalysis of randomised trials of antiplatelet therapy for prevention of death, myocardial infarction, and stroke in high-risk patients. BMJ. 2002;324:71–86.
59. The RISC Group. Risk of myocardial infarction and death during treatment with low dose aspirin and intravenous heparin in men with unstable coronary artery disease. Lancet. 1990;336:827–30.
60. Klimt CR, Knatterud GI, Stamler J, Meier P. Persantineaspirin reinfarction study II. Secondary coronary prevention with persantine and aspirin. J Am Coll Cardiol. 1986;7:251–69.
61. Sabatine MS, Cannon CP, Gibson CM, et al. Addition of clopidogrel to aspirin and fibrinolytic therapy for myocardial infarction with ST-segment elevation. N Engl J Med. 2005;352(12):1179–89.
62. Peters RJ, Mehta SR, Fox KA, et al. Effects of aspirin dose when used alone or in combination with clopidogrel in patients with acute coronary syndromes: observations from the Clopidogrel in Unstable angina to prevent Recurrent Events (CURE) study. Circulation. 2003;108(14):1682 7.
63. Steinhubl SR, Berger PB, Mann JT, et al. Early and sustained dual oral antiplatelet therapy following percutaneous coronary intervention a randomized controlled trial. JAMA. 2002;288:2411–20.
64. Jolly SS, Pogue J, Haladyn K, Peters RJ. Effects of aspirin dose on ischaemic events and bleeding after percutaneous coronary intervention: insights from the PCI-CURE study. Eur Heart J. 2009;30(8):900–7.
65. Wiviott S, Braunwald E, McCabe C, et al. Prasugrel versus clopidogrel in patients with acute coronary syndromes. N Engl J Med. 2007;357:2001–15.
66. Wallentin L, Becker RC, Budaj A, et al. Ticagrelor versus clopidogrel in patients with acute coronary syndromes. N Engl J Med. 2009;361:1045–57.
67. Cannon C, Harrington R, James S, et al. Ticagrelor compared with clopidogrel in acute coronary syndromes patients with a planned invasive strategy (PLATO): a randomized double-blind study. Lancet. 2010;375:283–93.

68. Sabatine MS, Cannon CP, Gibson CM, et al. Effect of clopidogrel pretreatment before percutaneous coronary intervention in patients with ST-elevation myocardial infarction treated with fibrinolytics: the PCI-CLARITY study. JAMA. 2005;294(10):1224–32.
69. The CURRENT-OASIS 7 Investigators. Dose comparisons of clopidogrel and aspirin in acute coronary syndromes. N Engl J Med. 2010;363:930–42.
70. Diener HC, Bogousslavsky J, Brass LM, et al. Aspirin and clopidogrel compared with clopidogrel alone after recent ischaemic stroke or transient ischaemic attack in high-risk patients (MATCH): randomised, double-blind, placebo-controlled trial. Lancet. 2004;364(9431):331–7.
71. Bhatt DL, Fox KA, Hacke W, et al. Clopidogrel and aspirin versus aspirin alone for the prevention of atherothrombotic events. N Engl J Med. 2006;354(16):1706–17.
72. CAPRIE Steering Committee. A randomised, blinded, trial of clopidogrel versus aspirin in patients at risk of ischaemic events (CAPRIE). CAPRIE Steering Committee. Lancet. 1996;348(9038):1329–39.
73. Yu X, Chen F, He J, et al. Duration of dual antiplatelet therapy after implantation of the first-generation and second-generation drug-eluting stents. Coron Artery Dis. 2013;24(3):217–23.
74. Public Health Advisory: Updated safety information about a drug interaction between Clopidogrel Bisulfate (marketed as Plavix) and Omeprazole (marketed as Prilosec and Prilosec OTC). Available at: http://www.fda.gov/Drugs/DrugSafety/PublicHealthAdvisories/ucm190825.htm. Accessed 28 May 2010.
75. Lau WC, Waskell LA, Watkins PB, et al. Atorvastatin reduces the ability of clopidogrel to inhibit platelet aggregation: a new drug-drug interaction. Circulation. 2003;107:32–7.
76. Neubauer HB, Günesdogan B, Hanefeld C, et al. Lipophilic statins interfere with the inhibitory effects of clopidogrel on platelet function: a flow cytometry study. Eur Heart. 2004;24:1744–9.
77. Piorkowski M, Weikert U, Schwimmbeck PL, et al. ADP induced platelet degranulation in healthy individuals is reduced by clopidogrel after pretreatment with atorvastatin. Thromb Haemost. 2004;92:614–20.
78. Mega JL, Close SL, Wiviott SD, et al. Cytochrome p-450 polymorphisms and response to clopidogrel. N Engl J Med. 2009;360:354–62.
79. Nguyen T, Frishman WH, Nawarskas J, et al. Variability of response to clopidogrel: possible mechanisms and clinical implications. Cardiol Rev. 2006;14:136–42.
80. Simon T, Verstuyft C, Mary-Krause M, et al. Genetic determinants of response to clopidogrel and cardiovascular events. N Engl J Med. 2009;360:363–75.

81. Abraham NS, Hlatky MA, Antman EM, et al. ACCF/ACG/AHA 2010 expert consensus document on the concomitant use of proton pump inhibitors and thienopyridines: a focused update of the ACCF/ACG/AHA 2008 expert consensus document on reducing the gastrointestinal risks of antiplatelet therapy and NSAID use. A Report of the American College of Cardiology Foundation Task Force on Expert Consensus Documents. J Am Coll Cardiol. 2010;56(24):2051–66.
82. Douglas IJ, Evans SJW, Hingorani AD, et al. Clopidogrel and interaction with proton pump inhibitors: comparison between cohort and within person study design. BMJ. 2012;345:e4388.
83. O'Donoghue ML, Braunwald E, Antman EM, et al. Pharmacodynamic effect and clinical efficacy of clopidogrel and prasugrel with or without a proton-pump inhibitor: an analysis of two randomised trials. Lancet. 2009;374(9694):989–97.
84. Topol EJ, GUSTO V Investigators. Reperfusion therapy for acute myocardial infarction with fibrinolytic therapy or combination reduced fibrinolytic therapy and platelet glycoprotein IIb/IIIa inhibition: the GUSTO V randomised trial. Lancet. 2001;357(9272):1905–14.
85. Assessment of the Safety and Efficacy of a New Thrombolytic Regimen (ASSENT)-3 Investigators. Efficacy and safety of tenecteplase in combination with enoxaparin, abciximab, or unfractionated heparin: the ASSENT-3 randomised trial in acute myocardial infarction. Lancet. 2001;358(9282):605–13.
86. De Luca G, Navarese E, Marino P. Risk profile and benefits from Gp IIb-IIIa inhibitors among patients with ST-segment elevation myocardial infarction treated with primary angioplasty: a meta-regression analysis of randomized trials. Eur Heart J. 2009;30:2705–13.
87. Ellis SG, Tendera M, de Belder MA, et al. Facilitated PCI in patients with ST-elevation myocardial infarction. N Engl J Med. 2008;358:2205–17.
88. Mehilli J, Kastrati A, Schulz S, Frungel S, et al. Abciximab in patients with acute ST-segment-elevation myocardial infarction undergoing primary percutaneous coronary intervention after clopidogrel loading: a randomized double-blind trial. Circulation. 2009;119:1933–40.
89. Lee CJ, Ansell JE. Direct rhombin inhibitors. B J Clin Pharm. 2011;72(4):581.
90. Bates SM, Weitz JI. The mechanism of action of thrombin inhibitors. J Invasive Cardiol. 2000;12(Suppl F):27F–32.
91. Giraldez RR, Nicolau JC, Corbalan R, et al. Enoxaparin is superior to unfractionated heparin in patients with ST elevation myocardial infarction undergoing fibrinolysis regardless of the choice of lytic: an ExTRACT-TIMI 25 analysis. Eur Heart J. 2007;28:1566–73.
92. Yusuf S, Mehta SR, Chrolavicius S, et al. Effects of fondaparinux on mortality and reinfarction in patients with acute ST-segment elevation myocardial infarction: the OASIS-6 randomized trial. JAMA. 2006;295:1519–30.

93. Montalescot G, Zeymer U, Silvain J, et al. Intravenous enoxaparin or unfractionated heparin in primary percutaneous coronary intervention for ST-elevation myocardial infarction: the international randomised open-label ATOLL trial. Lancet. 2011;378:693–703.
94. Mehran R, Lansky AJ, Witzenbichler B, et al. Bivalirudin in patients undergoing primary angioplasty for acute myocardial infarction (HORIZONS-AMI): 1-year results of a randomised controlled trial. Lancet. 2009;374:1149–59.
95. Andreotti F, Testa L, Biondi-Zoccai GGL, Crea F. Aspirin plus warfarin compared with aspirin alone after acute coronary syndromes: an up-dated and comprehensive meta-analysis. Eur Heart J. 2006;27:519–26.
96. Willoughby S, Holmes A, Loscalzo J. Platelets and cardiovascular disease. Eur J Cardiovasc Nurs. 2002;1(4):273–88.
97. Altman R. Risk factors in coronary atherosclerosis athero-inflammation: the meeting point. Thromb J. 2003;1(1):4.

Chapter 6
Triple Therapy: Risky but Sometimes Necessary

Rikke Sørensen and Gunnar Gislason

Introduction

Antithrombotic therapy is a cornerstone of treatment in various cardiovascular conditions, e.g. ischemic heart disease (IHD), atrial fibrillation (AF), artificial heart valves and stroke. The need for antithrombotic therapy in patients with cardiovascular disease can change over time due to temporal changes in patients baseline risk e.g. after stent implantation, insertion of an artificial heart valve, occurrence of venous thromboembolism or stroke. Hence, continuous evaluation of the patient's need for antithrombotic treatment is required, and treatments should be modified accordingly by changing to an alternative or more effective antithrombotic drug or combination of two or more drugs if indicated. Antithrombotic treatment is associated with increased risk of bleeding, a risk that is accentuated with combinational use, the highest

R. Sørensen, MD, PhD (✉)
Department of Cardiology,
Copenhagen University Hospital Bispebjerg,
Bispebjerg Bakke 23, København NV 2400, Denmark
e-mail: rs@heart.dk

G. Gislason, MD, PhD
Department of Cardiology,
Copenhagen University Hospital Gentofte, Hellerup, Denmark

P. Avanzas, P. Clemmensen (eds.), *Pharmacological Treatment of Acute Coronary Syndromes*, Current Cardiovascular Therapy,
DOI 10.1007/978-1-4471-5424-2_6,
© Springer-Verlag London 2014

risk being associated with triple treatment (consisting of oral anticoagulation, aspirin and a $P2Y_{12}$ inhibitor). Thus, bleeding risk assessment is an essential part of selecting the most appropriate antithrombotic treatment regimen for the individual patient [1, 2].

Most randomized trials exploring treatments with antithrombotic medications have included patients with a unanimous indication for antithrombotic treatment such as atrial fibrillation or acute coronary syndrome, and have assessed efficacy and safety in that given clinical setting [3–8]. However, everyday practice is challenged since patients often have more than one indication for antithrombotic treatment (e.g. atrial fibrillation *and* acute coronary syndrome) followed by a short or long-standing need for combining antithrombotic treatments that have mostly been tested separately. Knowledge of safety and efficacy of combinations with triple antithrombotic therapy is sparse primarily described by observational studies, or in smaller randomized trials [2, 9–11]. Continuous evaluation of the appropriateness of current antithrombotic treatment is highly important; especially in patients treated with triple therapy since patients experiencing a bleeding episode have a poorer prognosis with increased risk of thrombosis and death [12, 13].

On the basis of present literature this chapter will describe clinical situations in which combinations of oral anticoagulation and antiplatelet therapy are needed after discharge from hospital. The safety and risks related to different combinations of triple therapy and the alternative dual therapy will be reviewed. In addition we will point out the acknowledged tools to assessment of individual risk of bleeding and everyday handling.

Ischemic Heart Disease

Acute Coronary Syndrome

Acute coronary syndrome occurs when there is an unstable plaque in the coronary artery, leading to a subtotal or total occlusion. The process of thrombus-formation is accelerated by activated platelets and activation of the coagulation cascade. The immediate antithrombotic treatment of acute coronary syndrome includes loading dose with aspirin and a $P2Y_{12}$ inhibitor (clopidogrel, ticagrelor or prasugrel), along with anticoagulant treatment (typically fondaparinux, or low-molecular weight heparins) until invasive examination and revascularization are possible [14, 15]. Long-term antithrombotic treatment after the initial phase of the acute coronary syndrome is based on dual antiplatelet therapy (aspirin and a $P2Y_{12}$ inhibitor) [14, 15].In the Clopidogrel in Unstable Angina to Prevent Recurrent Events (CURE) trial treatment with clopidogrel and aspirin were found to be superior to aspirin monotherapy considering a combined endpoint of cardiovascular death and non-fatal myocardial infarction (MI) or stroke, and also recurrent MI alone [3]. However, several studies have shown that clopidogrel have some disadvantages, primarily that up to 40 % of the patients have insufficient inhibition of the platelets if treated with clopidogrel (clopidogrel resistance) [16, 17]. This variance is caused by several factors: genetic variations, drug-drug interactions and poor adherence to treatment. Several assays have been developed to identify patients with clopidogrel resistance, but the assays have yet not been proved usable in everyday clinical practice, primarily due to diversity of sensitivity and difficulties by determining a relevant cut-off value [18–20]. Prasugrel and ticagrelor have proven to be more effective than clopidogrel in acute coronary syndrome, with a lower degree of variation to platelet inhibition [21, 22]. Prasugrel is activated by one-step of hepatic activation, whereas clopidogrel is activated by a two-step process, and ticagrelor binds directly and reversible to the $P2Y_{12}$ inhibitor. The Trial to Assess Improvement in Therapeutic Outcomes by Optimizing Platelet Inhibition with Prasugrel–Thrombolysis in Myocardial Infarction (TRITON–TIMI) 38explored dual therapy with prasugrel and aspirin against dual therapy with clopidogrel and aspirin and found reduced frequency of the combined endpoint of recurrent MI, cardiovascular death and non-fatal stroke, primarily driven by reduction of recurrent MI and cardiovascular death [5].In the Study of Platelet inhibition and Patient Outcomes (PLATO) trial ticagrelor and aspirin reduced a composed endpoint of cardiovascular or cerebrovascular death and recurrent MI compared with the combination of clopidogrel and aspirin [4]. The CURE, TRITON-TIMI 38, and PLATO trials tested dual-antiplatelet therapy in the setting of acute coronary syndrome. All studies excluded patients with an indication of anticoagulation [3–5]. Nevertheless, approximately 6–8 % of the patients being admitted with acute coronary syndrome have an indication for oral anticoagulation, whereas it is estimated that 20–30 % of patients with AF with an indication of oral anticoagulation have co-existing coronary artery disease. Consequently, the need for combining dual-antiplatelet therapy and oral anticoagulation (triple therapy) is overt [14, 23].

Percutaneous Coronary Intervention

In patients treated with percutaneous coronary intervention (PCI) stent-thrombosis is a feared complication, since it often is fatal [24]. The frequency of stent-thrombosis, both early and late is higher in patients treated with first-generation drug-eluting stents compared with bare-metal stents [25, 26]. Early discontinuation of treatment with a $P2Y_{12}$ inhibitor has shown to be the strongest independent predictor of stent-thrombosis [27]. The optimal duration of dual antiplatelet therapy has been debated and tested, but beneficial effect of clopidogrel treatment beyond 12 month seem to be out-weighed by increased risk of bleeding [28–30]. Since 2010, the recommended duration of dual antiplatelet treatment after PCI (without MI) is 1–3 months for bare metal stents, and 6–12 months for drug-eluting stents, the variation in length of therapy to be adjusted according to the patients risk of bleeding (details on bleeding risk assessment is listed below) [14, 15, 23].

Indications for Oral Anticoagulation

The risk of stroke in patients with AF is increased with presence of comorbidities and age. Risk stratification is easily assessed by e.g. CHA_2DS_2VASc risk score (Congestive heart failure or left ventricular dysfunction, hypertension, Age ≥75(doubled), Diabetes, Stroke (doubled), Vascular disease, Age 65–74, Sex category (female)). In patients with no contraindications oral anticoagulation is recommended in patients with CHA_2DS_2VASc score ≥1 (except for patients at low risk achieving 1 point for female gender), since treatment with aspirin monotherapy and dual therapy of aspirin and clopidogrel is less effective regarding stroke prevention [31, 32].In patients with other conditions e.g. pulmonary embolism or prosthetic heart valves oral anticoagulation can be necessary for a limited period of time or lifelong, to reduce the risk of stroke or recurrent embolism [33–38], sometimes in combination with aspirin [39].

Triple Therapy

Triple therapy defined by use of aspirin, a $P2Y_{12}$ inhibitor and oral anticoagulation can be indicated in certain clinical situations but usually for a limited period of time. The typical clinical situation: a patient with a clear indication of oral anticoagulation experiencing an acute MI or is treated with a coronary stent. The following sections will cover description and discussion of safety and risks related to different combinations of triple therapy and an alternative dual therapy. Both oral anticoagulation with vitamin K antagonists and the novel oral anticoagulants will be reviewed.

Triple Therapy: Aspirin, Clopidogrel and Vitamin K Antagonist

Bleedings

Several studies have described the risk of bleeding and the risk of thromboses related to triple therapy, mainly in combination of vitamin K antagonist treatment, aspirin and clopidogrel treatment. However, these studies are difficult to compare directly due to diverse populations (stable and unstable patients, difference in age and severity of comorbidity), and use of different definitions of bleeding. In general, the studies have found higher risk of bleeding related to triple therapy (vitamin K antagonist, aspirin and clopidogrel) compared with mono- and dual-therapy; the crude incidences of major bleedings ranging between 5 and 15 %, mostly being >10 % per year [1, 2, 9, 10, 40–42]. It has been more difficult to establish concordance of bleeding risk related to dual antithrombotic treatment with a vitamin K antagonist and either aspirin or clopidogrel [1, 9, 10, 40, 42, 43]. Treatment with the combination of vitamin K antagonist and clopidogrel have previously been recommended and considered safe, in patients with high risk of bleeding needing triple therapy [44, 45]. A statement that was challenged by two large scale nationwide observational studies, which found nearly comparable risk of bleeding with dual treatment of vitamin K antagonists and clopidogrel as with triple therapy [1, 42]. Recently the results of the What is the Optimal antiplatelet and anticoagulant therapy in patients with oral anticoagulation and coronary StenTing (WOEST) trial were published and to our knowledge, this is the first randomized trial testing safety of triple therapy against dual treatment with vitamin K antagonist and clopidogrel. A total of 573 patients treated with PCI, with an indication of OAC were included. The study was powered to test difference in risk of bleeding with a follow-up of 1 year. The study clearly showed reduced risk of bleeding in patients receiving vitamin k antagonist treatment combined with clopidogrel compared with triple therapy (6.5 % vs. 12.7 %, p = 0.01, Bleeding Academy Research Consort definition, type 3 bleeding). Results persisted across subgroups, but due to low number of patients in each subgroup the results did not reach significance in all. The numbers of cerebral-bleedings were comparable in both the triple and dual treatment group (1.1 %). The incidences of bleeding in the study was relatively high (triple therapy 15.8 %, vitamin K antagonist and clopidogrel 6.5 %), but not markedly different from real-life patients in large observational studies [1, 2, 42, 46]. The previously found high risk of bleeding related to the combinations of vitamin K antagonists and clopidogrel in the observational studies may be explained by selection bias (patients at higher risk was selected for a presumed safer antithrombotic strategy), emphasizing the importance of randomized trials to guide clinical practice [1, 42, 46]. Noteworthy, the WOEST trial found reduced all-cause mortality in the group treated with vitamin K antagonists and clopidogrel. One could speculate that this could be due to a lower number of bleedings, as a bleeding occurrence is followed by at higher risk of thrombosis and death [2]. Table 6.1 shows different studies and crude incidences of bleeding related to treatment with vitamin k antagonist in combination with one or two antiplatelet treatments.

Thrombosis

There are no randomized studies of patients in treatment with oral anticoagulation in combination with one or two antiplatelet drugs that have been powered to test frequency of mortality and stent thrombosis [15]. Two observational studies found comparable risk of thrombotic events among patients treated with triple therapy and vitamin K antagonist combined with one antiplatelet drug (aspirin or clopidogrel), but the thrombotic endpoints assessed were different, one being a combined endpoint, another being separate measurements of death, stroke, recurrent MI, or unscheduled PCI, the rates are therefore not directly comparable. None of the studies had the opportunity to evaluate stent-thrombosis [42, 43]. The WOEST trial was not powered to detect differences in rates of mortality or thrombosis (main interest being death, stent-thrombosis and recurrent MI), but the number of events were reassuring with an all-cause mortality of 2.5 and 6.3 %, for the dual and triple treatment group, respectively, p = 0.03. Recurrent MI, stroke, or stent-thrombosis not being numerical higher in the dual treatment group compared with the triple group [2]. Clearly, the European Society of Cardiology recommends thorough consideration of the antithrombotic regimen following PCI in patients with an indication for oral anticoagulation (both stable and acute patients)

TABLE 6.1 Bleeding incidences listed in different studies according to dual therapy or triple therapy (combinations of vitamin K antagonists, aspirin and clopidogrel)

Author	Design	n	% ACS	% PCI	VKA+ aspirin	VKA+ clopidogrel	VKA+ aspirin or clopidogrel[b]	Triple	Bleeding definition
Buresly et al. [40]	Observational	21,443	100 %	No data	8.3 %	6.8 %		8.3 %	Admission to a hospital with a bleeding diagnosis
Karjalainen et al. [9]	Observational	239	53.5 %	100 %	6.1 %	11.1 %		6.6 %	Major: decrease of blood hemoglobin level >4.0 g/dL, the need blood transfusion of >2 units, need for surgery, or intracranial/ retroperitoneal bleeding
Nguyen et al. [43]	Observational	800	100 %	34 %			4.6 %	5.9 %	GRACE definition, in-hospital bleedings

Ruiz-Nodar et al. [10]	Observational	426	83.9 %	100 %			14.9 %[c]	14.9 %[c]	Decrease of blood hemoglobin level >5.0 g/dL, the need blood transfusion of >2 units, need for surgery, or intracranial/retroperitoneal bleeding
Sørensen et al. [1]	Observational	40,812	100 %	37 %	5.1 %	12.3 %		12.0 %	Admission to a hospital with a bleeding diagnosis
Lamberts et al. [42]	Observational	11,480	76.4 %	23.6 %	9.5 %	10.6 %		14.2 %	Admission to a hospital with a bleeding diagnosis

(continued)

Table 6.1 (continued)

Author	Design	% ACS	% PCI	VKA+ aspirin	VKA+ clopidogrel	VKA+ aspirin or clopidogrel[b]	Triple	Bleeding definition
Hurlen et al. [41]	Randomized	3,560	100 %	36.5 %[a]	2.3 %				Major: nonfatal/fatal cerebral hemorrhage, bleeding needing surgical revision or blood transfusion.
Dewilde et al. [2]	Randomized	573	25 %	100 %		6.5 %		15.8 %	Bleeding Academy Research Consort, type 3

ACS acute coronary syndrome, *PCI* percutaneous coronary intervention, *VKA* vitamin K antagonist

[a]PCI or coronary artery bypass surgery

[b]Not specified if it was clopidogrel or aspirin

[c]Not differentiated whether the patient received one or two antiplatelet treatments

[14, 15, 23]. Presences/absence of acute coronary syndrome, individual assessment of bleeding risk, and type of stent are important factors when determining duration of triple therapy treatment. Bare-metal stent is preferred as stent choice in patients at high risk of bleeding (recommended 4 weeks of triple therapy). Drug-eluting stents can be used in patients with low or intermediate risk of bleeding, the '-ilumus' stents (sirolimus, everolimus, and tacrolimus) requires at least 3 months of triple therapy, the paclitaxel-eluting stent at least 6 months. These recommendations will probably be challenged in the future, as second-generation drug-eluting stents (everolimus-eluting stent) in a recent meta-analysis have be associated with a lower risk of stent thrombosis compared with first-generation drug-eluting-stents and bare-metal stents [31].

Triple Therapy: Aspirin, Clopidogrel and a Novel Anticoagulant Therapy

Triple therapy with rivaroxaban, apixaban, or dabigatran etexilate added on top of dual antiplatelet therapy with aspirin and clopidogrel, has been tested in patients with acute coronary syndrome, to explore whether a prolonged anticoagulation could reduce the residual risk of thrombosis in patients with MI [47–49]. Apixaban was added on top of aspirin and clopidogrel in therapeutic doses (5 mg b.i.d.), whereas rivaroxaban was used in lower dose than recommended for oral anticoagulation (2.5 mg or 5.0 mg daily). Dabigatran was tested in a phase II trial at different doses (50 mg, 75 mg, 110 mg, 150 mg b.i.d.) on top of aspirin and clopidogrel [47–49].

Rivaroxaban in Triple Therapy

The Anti-Xa Therapy to Lower Cardiovascular Eventsin Addition to Standard Therapy in Subjects with Acute Coronary Syndrome-Thrombolysis in Myocardial Infarction

51 (ATLAS ACS 2-TIMI 51) included 15,526 acute coronary syndrome patients randomized to the following treatments: (1) Aspirin and clopidogrel, (2) Aspirin, clopidogrel, and rivaroxaban 2.5 mg daily, (3) Aspirin, clopidogrel, and rivaroxaban 5 mg daily. The lower dose of rivaroxaban was chosen, since a phase-2 dose-finding trial found dose-dependent increase of bleedings with higher doses of rivaroxaban, bleeding rates being: 20 mg 15.3 %, 15 mg 12.7 %, 10 mg 10.9 %, 5 mg 6.1 %, placebo 3.3 % [50]. Primary efficacy endpoint of the ATLAS ACS 2-TIMI 51 trial was a combined endpoint of cardiovascular death, myocardial infarction or stroke, the safety endpoint was major bleeding (TIMI-major bleeding definition). The mean duration of treatment with rivaroxaban was approximately 1 year. The outcome of the study was: reduced combined endpoint of cardiovascular death, myocardial infarction or stroke in the groups receiving rivaroxaban (8.9 % with combined rivaroxaban 2.5 and 5 mg, 10.7 % with placebo, $p = 0.008$). The safety endpoint was increased with TIMI-major bleedings of 2.1 % with combined rivaroxaban 2.5 and 5 mg, and 0.6 % with placebo, $p < 0.001$. Separate tests of 2.5 and 5 mg showed reduction of the combined efficacy endpoint ($p = 0.02$ and 0.03, respectively) and increased frequency of the safety endpoint ($p < 0.001$ for both), though the numbers of bleedings were numerically lower in the group receiving 2.5 mg rivaroxaban compared with 5 mg ($p = 0.12$). In addition, rivaroxaban 2.5 mg reduced all cause mortality [49].

Apixaban in Triple Therapy

The Apixaban for Prevention of Acute Ischemic Events 2 (APPRAISE-2)study explored in a population of patients with acute coronary syndrome, the efficacy and safety of apixaban 5 mg b.i.d. combined with either aspirin and clopidogrel or aspirin alone against dual antiplatelet therapy with aspirin and clopidogrel or aspirin monotherapy (pooled in one group). The primary efficacy endpoint was a combined of cardiovascular death, myocardial infarction or stroke, the safety endpoint major bleeding (TIMI-major definition).

Recruitment was planned to include 10,500 patients with acute coronary syndrome, but was stopped prematurely after randomization of approximately 7,000 patients, due to excess of bleedings in the apixaban group, without benefit on the efficacy endpoint. Among the patients included, with a mean follow-up of 240 days, the efficacy endpoint of cardiovascular death, myocardial infarction or stroke occurred in 7.5 and 7.9 % in the apixaban and placebo group, respectively (p = 0.51). The corresponding values for the safety endpoint were: 1.3 % in the apixaban group, and 0.5 % in the placebo group, p = 0.001, with more fatal, intracranial and clinical relevant non-major bleedings in the apixaban group [47].

Dabigatran in Triple Therapy

As for dabigatran, a phase III study in patients with acute coronary syndrome has not been initiated. Dabigatran tested on top of aspirin and clopidogrel in a Phase II trial lead to more bleedings among patients treated with dabigatran (dose dependent). The bleeding rates were: dabigatran 50 mg b.i.d 3.5 %, 75 mg b.i.d 4.3 %, 110 mg b.i.d 7.9 %, and 150 mg b.i.d 7.8 %, the bleedings defined as major and clinical relevant minor bleedings [48]. A subgroup analysis of the Randomized Evaluation of Long-Term Anticoagulation Therapy (RE-LY) study was performed to test whether the safety and efficacy of dabigatran was affected by concomitant antiplatelet therapy (which was used in 38.4 % of the included patients at some point during the study-period) [51]. The population in the RE-LY study consisted of AF patients, the primary efficacy endpoint being stroke or systemic embolism, the safety endpoint being bleeding. The main results of the subgroup analysis confirmed the results from the main analysis that dabigatran 110 mg b.i.d. was non-inferior to warfarin, with less bleedings irrespective of concomitant antiplatelet use. In patients with dabigatran 150 mg the efficacy endpoint occurred less in patients without antiplatelet therapy, with a reduced benefit among those taking antiplatelet therapy (p for interaction = 0.06). Overall, the safety endpoint was similar in patients with dabigatran 150 mg and warfarin irrespective of antiplatelet use. Since use of antiplatelet therapy changed during the studyperiod the analyses of safety was also tested time-dependently, showing increased risk of bleeding associated with antiplatelet use, a risk that was accentuated with the number of antiplatelets used (HR 2.31; CI 1.79–2.98 for dual-antiplatelet, HR 1.60; CI 1.42–1.82 for one antiplatelet, no antiplatelet as reference) [6, 51].

Triple Therapy, Summary and Discussion

Use of antiplatelet therapy in combination with oral anticoagulation can be necessary for limited time periods to prevent serious thrombotic events as stroke, recurrent MI, stent-thrombosis, and death. The treatment should be used only during the period of time where the risk of thrombosis is high, at present a maximum of 12 months is recommended for patients with an indication of oral anticoagulation experiencing a MI (Table 6.2) [14, 15, 52, 53]. Combinational use of oral anticoagulation and antiplatelet therapy increases the risk of bleeding, both when considering triple therapy with vitamin k antagonists, aspirin and clopidogrel and triple therapy with a novel anticoagulant: rivaroxaban, apixaban or dabigatran in combination with aspirin and clopidogrel. Increased number of drugs accentuates the risk of bleeding, as does increased doses of a novel anticoagulant drug [1, 42, 47–51]. Occurrence of a bleeding is followed by an increased risk of thromboses and death, which might explain the beneficial effect on all cause mortality of low dose rivaroxaban (2.5 mg) in combination with aspirin and clopidogrel, but not in the high doses, and the reduced mortality found in the WOEST trial among patients receiving vitamin K antagonist and clopidogrel, compared with patients in triple therapy.

In clinical settings where triple therapy is indicated combinations of vitamin K antagonist or dabigatran 110 mg, aspirin and clopidogrel can be used [14, 15, 51–53]. Rivaroxaban has not been tested in combination with aspirin and clopidogrel in doses recommended for e.g. AF or pulmonary embolism, since the doses of rivaroxaban used in the ATLAS-ACS

TABLE 6.2 Incidences of thrombosis, revascularisation or death listed in different studies according to dual therapy or triple therapy (combinations of vitamin K antagonists, aspirin and clopidogrel)

Author	Design	n	% ACS	% PCI	VKA+ aspirin	VKA+ clopidogrel	VKA+ aspirin or clopidogrel[a]	Triple	Thrombotic event
Karjalainen et al. [9]	Observational	239	53.5 %	100 %	15.2 %	0 %		1.9 %	Death/stent thrombosis
Nguyen et al. [43]	Observational	800	100 %	34 %	–	–	12.0 %/0 %	7.4 %/3.2 %	Death/MI
Ruiz-Nodar et al. [10]	Observational	426	83.5 %	100 %	–	–	17.8 %/1.3 %[b]	17.8 %/1.3 %[b]	Death/stent thrombosis
Lamberts et al. [42]	Observational	11,480	76.4 %	23.6 %	–	–	19.4 %	20.1 %	Cardiovascular death/MI/stroke
Dewilde et al. [2]	Randomized	573	25 %	100 %	–	2.5 %/1.4 %	–	6.3 %/3.2 %	Death/stent thrombosis

ACS acute coronary syndrome, *PCI* percutaneous coronary intervention, *VKA* vitamin K antagonist, *MI* myocardial infarction

[a]Not specified if it was aspirin or clopidogrel

[b]Not differentiated whether the patient received one or two antiplatelet treatments

2-TIMI 51 study was reduced (2.5 and 5 mg) [49]. Triple therapy with apixaban, aspirin, and clopidogrel cannot be recommended at present since an increased risk of bleeding was found in the APPRAISE-2 study (when compared with dual treatment of aspirin and clopidogrel), however it is currently unknown whether this risk is higher than other combinations of triple therapy since no study has made direct comparison [47]. Results from the WOEST trial indicates that dual-therapy with vitamin K antagonists is associated with reduced risk of bleeding, without increased risk of thrombosis. Unfortunately the study was not powered to detected difference in thrombotic events e.g. stent-thrombosis, but the results are reassuring and support that dual therapy with clopidogrel and vitamin K-antagonist can be used as a safer combination in patients at high risk of bleeding [2, 52]. At present, there are no published studies available addressing the combinational use of oral anticoagulation, aspirin and the newer $P2Y_{12}$ inhibitors prasugrel and ticagrelor, thus the efficacy and safety of these combinations is currently unknown and cannot be recommended.

Triple Therapy in Everyday Care

Assessment of Bleeding Risk: Different Bleeding Risk Schemes

Individual assessment of bleeding risk is important every time an antithrombotic treatment is initiated, since bleeding is known to increase risk of recurrent thrombosis and death [1, 12]. Several risk schemes have been developed in patients with AF [54–56] and patients with acute coronary syndrome [57, 58], assessing both in-hospital bleeding and long-term bleeding. Some of the validated risk scores for AF are: (1) the HAS-BLED risk score (Hypertension, Abnormal Renal/Liver Function, Stroke, Bleeding History or Predisposition, Labile International Normalized Ratio, Elderly, Drugs/Alcohol), (2) the HEMORR(2)HAGES risk score (Hepatic or Renal Disease, Ethanol Abuse, Malignancy,

Older Age, Reduced Platelet Count or Function, Re-Bleeding, Hypertension, Anemia, Genetic Factors, Excessive Fall Risk and Stroke), and (3) the ATRIA risk score (Anticoagulation and Risk Factors in Atrial Fibrillation) [54–56]. The risk scores for patients with acute coronary syndrome are: (1) The GRACE score (the Global Registry of Acute Coronary Events), and (2) The CRUSADE risk score (Can Rapid Risk Stratification of Unstable Angina Patients Suppress Adverse Outcomes with Early Implementation of ACC/AHA Guidelines) [57, 58]. The risk-schemes are based on individual risk factors associated with increased bleeding risk, the strongest ones being age, renal failure, and previous bleeding [54, 57–59]. Differences in the predictive values of the risk schemes have been estimated. In patients with AF the HAS-BLED risk score has shown to be superior compared with HEMORR(2)HAGES, and ATRIA [59, 60]. In patients with acute coronary syndrome no difference of the predictive value of the CRUSADADE and the GRACE risk scores was found [61]. In the guidelines of management of AF and patients with acute coronary syndrome it is recommended that individual bleeding risk is assessed, recommending the HAS-BLED score in AF patients, but without a direct recommendation of one risk score in patients with acute coronary syndrome [14, 15, 53]. In general, bleeding risk scores should be considered as an objective clinical tool, which can be helpful in selecting the most appropriate antithrombotic regimen for a given clinical situation [14, 23].

Additional Proton-Pump Inhibitors?

The use of proton-pump inhibitors (PPIs) in acute coronary syndrome have been debated heavily. It has been suspected that interaction with clopidogrel during inhibition of the cytochrome P2C19 system could reduce the inhibition of the platelets and thus increase the risk of serious thromboembolic events [62]. PPIs are used in approximately 30 % of patients with ACS [63, 64], thus great effort has been made to explore this question. Analyses of both observational studies and randomized trials have shown comparable risk of thrombotic events among those treated with or without PPIs while receiving a $P2Y_{12}$ inhibitor (clopidogrel or prasugrel) [63–65]. In a randomized trial of patients with an indication of dual antiplatelet therapy testing omeprazol towards placebo, found that omeprazol reduced gastrointestinal bleeding from 2.9 to 1.1 %, $p < 0.001$ [65]. The strongest predictors of upper gastrointestinal bleeding are: use of NSAIDs, steroids, oral anticoagulation, previous gastrointestinal bleeding, and patients with helicobacter pylori infection [66, 67].It is recommended that at least patients with these characteristics should receive concomitant PPIs while taking antithrombotic medications as gastric protection, especially if the treatment counts more than one antithrombotic drug [14, 15, 23].

Level of INR

Variance of the International Normalized Ratio (INR) values in patients treated with vitamin K antagonists is a predictor of increased risk of bleeding (INR >2.6) [23]. Based on two smaller studies it is recommended in AF patients treated with vitamin K antagonist and dual antiplatelet therapy that target INR is kept between 2.0 and 2.5 (Class IIa, evidence level c) [23, 68, 69]. Considering the results from the WOEST trial, patients that are difficult to keep within INR 2.0–2.5 could be considered candidates for a reduced dual antithrombotic therapy regimen with vitamin K antagonist treatment combined with clopidogrel. Although this was not directly studied in the WOEST trial the safety of this regimen was reassuring [2].

Duration of Triple Therapy

Bleeding risk is clearly increased with triple therapy, thus it is highly important to minimize exposure to triple therapy and keep the treatment period as short as possible. Recommended treatment length is dependent on presence/absence of acute coronary syndrome, risk of bleeding and type of stent used in patients treated with PCI. Table 6.3 shows recommendation set by the European Society of Cardiology [23]. In general, bleedings occur early after initiation of triple therapy. In the WOEST trial most bleedings occurred within 180 days, and a Danish study exploring the timing of bleeding showed the

TABLE 6.3 Recommended antithrombotic strategies following coronary artery s tenting in patients with AF in which oral anticoagulation is required

Haemorrhagic risk	Clinical setting	Stent implanted	Recommendations
Low or intermediate	Elective	Bare metal	1 month: triple therapy of warfarin (INR 2.0–2.5) + aspirin ≤100 mg/day + clopidogrel 75 mg/day
			Lifelong: warfarin (INR 2.0–3.0) alone
	Elective	Drug eluting	3 (–olimus group) to 6 (paclitaxel) months: triple therapy of warfarin (INR 2.0–2.5) + aspirin ≤100 mg/day + clopidogrel 75 mg/day
			Up to 12 months: combination of warfarin (INR 2.0–2.5) + clopidogrel 75 mg/day (or aspirin 100 mg/day)[a]
			Lifelong: warfarin (INR 2.0–3.0) alone
	ACS	Bare metal/ drug eluting	6 months: triple therapy of warfarin (INR 2.0–2.5) + aspirin ≤100 mg/day + clopidogrel 75 mg/day
			Up to 12 months: combination of warfarin (INR 2.0–2.5) + clopidogrel 75 mg/day (or aspirin 100 mg/day)[a]
			Lifelong: warfarin (INR 2.0–3.0) alone

(continued)

TABLE 6.3 (continued)

Haemorrhagic risk	Clinical setting	Stent implanted	Recommendations
High	Elective	Bare metal[b]	2–4 weeks: triple therapy of warfarin (INR 2.0–2.5) + aspirin ≤100 mg/day + clopidogrel 75 mg/day
			Lifelong: warfarin (INR 2.0–3.0) alone
	ACS	Bare metal[b]	4 weeks: triple therapy of warfarin (INR 2.0–2.5) + aspirin ≤100 mg/day + clopidogrel 75 mg/day
			Up to 12 months: combination of warfarin (INR 2.0–2.5) + clopidogrel 75 mg/day (or aspirin 100 mg/day); mg/day)[a]
			Lifelong: warfarin (INR 2.0–3.0) alone

Printed with permission from *European Heart Journal*
INK international normalized ratio, *ACS* acute coronary syndrome
[a]Combination of warfarin (INK 2.0–2.5) + aspirin ≤100 mg/day may be considered as an alternative
[b]Drug-eluting stents should be avoided

highest risk of bleeding during the first 90 days, but with a bleeding incidence of >10 % the first 180 days [2, 42]. Estimating baseline risk of bleeding before initiation of triple therapy is warranted, along with concurrent initiation of gastric protection with PPIs. In addition a planned determination of triple treatment according to recommendations should be set, to avoid inappropriate prolonged therapy. Figure 6.1 provides a checklist of considerations before initiating triple therapy in a patient.

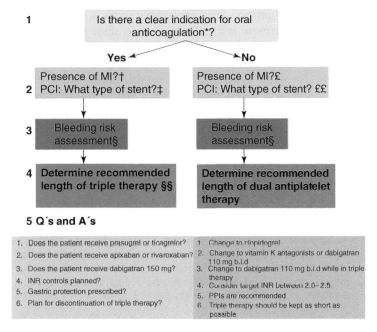

1 **Is there a clear indication for oral anticoagulation*?**

Yes / No

Presence of MI?†
2 **PCI: What type of stent?‡** | **Presence of MI?£**
PCI: What type of stent? ££

3 **Bleeding risk assessment§** | **Bleeding risk assessment§**

4 **Determine recommended length of triple therapy §§** | **Determine recommended length of dual antiplatelet therapy**

5 Q´s and A´s

1. Does the patient receive prasugrel or ticagrelor?	1. Change to clopidogrel
2. Does the patient receive apixaban or rivaroxaban?	2. Change to vitamin K antagonists or dabigatran 110 mg b.i.d
3. Does the patient receive dabigatran 150 mg?	3. Change to dabigatran 110 mg b.i.d while in triple therapy
4. INR controls planned?	4. Consider target INR between 2.0–2.5
5. Gastric protection prescribed?	5. PPIs are recommended
6. Plan for discontinuation of triple therapy?	6. Triple therapy should be kept as short as possible

* Most common indications for oral anticoagulation are: AF**, venous thromboembolism, prosthetic heart valves.
**Evaluation of thrombotic risk in AF patients by e.g. CHA₂DS₂VASc-score: oral anticoagulation is usually recommended for CHA₂ DS₂ VASc ≥1 (unless if 1 point is for female sex).
†Triple therapy is recommended for 1-12 months depending on the risk of bleeding §§
††Without MI: bare metal stent 1 months triple therapy, drug-eluting stents 3-6 months triple therapy (depending stent -type). With MI 1-12 months triple therapy depending n stenttype and bleeding risk §§
§ Evaluation by use of a bleeding risk scheme e.g. HAS-BLED, CRUSADE bleeding risk, if high bleeding risk consider dual treatment with oral anticoagulation and clopidogrel
§§Use Table 3 for guidance
£ Dual antiplatelet therapy for 12 month
££ Dual antiplatelet therapy for 1-12 month depending on stenttype.

FIGURE 6.1 Everyday care: checklist when you consider triple therapy

Conclusions

Triple therapy with dual antiplatelet therapy and oral anticoagulation can be indicated in certain clinical situations, usually for a limited period of time to prevent serious thrombotic events. Triple therapy increases the risk of bleeding, and continuous evaluation of the appropriateness of current anti-thrombotic treatment is highly important, since patients who experience a bleeding have a poorer prognosis. Recommended duration of triple therapy is dependent on presence/absence of acute coronary syndrome, risk of bleeding and type of stent used in patients treated with PCI. Triple therapy should be kept as short as possible, and include oral anticoagulation of vitamin K antagonist or dabigatran 110 mg b.i.d, aspirin, and clopidogrel.

References

1. Sorensen R, Hansen ML, Abildstrom SZ, Hvelplund A, Andersson C, Jorgensen C, et al. Risk of bleeding in patients with acute myocardial infarction treated with different combinations of aspirin, clopidogrel, and vitamin K antagonists in Denmark: a retrospective analysis of nationwide registry data. Lancet. 2009;374(9706): 1967–74.
2. Dewilde WJ, Oirbans T, Verheugt FW, Kelder JC, De Smet BJ, Herrman JP, et al. Use of clopidogrel with or without aspirin in patients taking oral anticoagulant therapy and undergoing percutaneous coronary intervention: an open-label, randomised, controlled trial. Lancet. 2013;381:1107–15.
3. Yusuf S, Zhao F, Mehta SR, Chrolavicius S, Tognoni G, Fox KK. Effects of clopidogrel in addition to aspirin in patients with acute coronary syndromes without ST-segment elevation. N Engl J Med. 2001;345(7):494–502.
4. Wallentin L, Becker RC, Budaj A, Cannon CP, Emanuelsson H, Held C, et al. Ticagrelor versus clopidogrel in patients with acute coronary syndromes. N Engl J Med. 2009;361(11):1045–57.
5. Wiviott SD, Braunwald E, McCabe CH, Montalescot G, Ruzyllo W, Gottlieb S, et al. Prasugrel versus clopidogrel in patients with acute coronary syndromes. N Engl J Med. 2007;357(20):2001–15.
6. Connolly SJ, Ezekowitz MD, Yusuf S, Eikelboom J, Oldgren J, Parekh A, et al. Dabigatran versus warfarin in patients with atrial fibrillation. N Engl J Med. 2009;361(12):1139–51.
7. Granger CB, Alexander JH, McMurray JJ, Lopes RD, Hylek EM, Hanna M, et al. Apixaban versus warfarin in patients with atrial fibrillation. N Engl J Med. 2011;365(11):981–92.
8. Patel MR, Mahaffey KW, Garg J, Pan G, Singer DE, Hacke W, et al. Rivaroxaban versus warfarin in nonvalvular atrial fibrillation. N Engl J Med. 2011;365(10):883–91.

9. Karjalainen PP, Porela P, Ylitalo A, Vikman S, Nyman K, Vaittinen MA, et al. Safety and efficacy of combined antiplatelet-warfarin therapy after coronary stenting. Eur Heart J. 2007;28(6):726–32.

10. Ruiz-Nodar JM, Marin F, Hurtado JA, Valencia J, Pinar E, Pineda J, et al. Anticoagulant and antiplatelet therapy use in 426 patients with atrial fibrillation undergoing percutaneous coronary intervention and stent implantation implications for bleeding risk and prognosis. J Am Coll Cardiol. 2008;51(8):818–25.

11. Jensen-Urstad K, Bouvier F, Hojer J, Ruiz H, Hulting J, Samad B, et al. Comparison of different echocardiographic methods with radionuclide imaging for measuring left ventricular ejection fraction during acute myocardial infarction treated by thrombolytic therapy. Am J Cardiol. 1998;81(5):538–44.

12. Rao SV, O'Grady K, Pieper KS, Granger CB, Newby LK, Van de Werf F, et al. Impact of bleeding severity on clinical outcomes among patients with acute coronary syndromes. Am J Cardiol. 2005;96(9):1200–6.

13. Eikelboom JW, Mehta SR, Anand SS, Xie C, Fox KA, Yusuf S. Adverse impact of bleeding on prognosis in patients with acute coronary syndromes. Circulation. 2006;114(8):774–82.

14. Hamm CW, Bassand JP, Agewall S, Bax J, Boersma E, Bueno H, et al. ESC Guidelines for the management of acute coronary syndromes in patients presenting without persistent ST-segment elevation: The Task Force for the management of acute coronary syndromes (ACS) in patients presenting without persistent ST-segment elevation of the European Society of Cardiology (ESC). Eur Heart J. 2011;32(23):2999–3054.

15. Steg PG, James SK, Atar D, Badano LP, Blomstrom-Lundqvist C, Borger MA, et al. ESC guidelines for the management of acute myocardial infarction in patients presenting with ST segment elevation. Eur Heart J. 2012;33(20):2569–619.

16. Gurbel PA, Bliden KP, Hiatt BL, O'Connor CM. Clopidogrel for coronary stenting: response variability, drug resistance, and the effect of pretreatment platelet reactivity. Circulation. 2003;107(23):2908–13.

17. Serebruany VL, Steinhubl SR, Berger PB, Malinin AI, Bhatt DL, Topol EJ. Variability in platelet responsiveness to clopidogrel among 544 individuals. J Am Coll Cardiol. 2005;45(2):246–51.

18. O'Donoghue M, Wiviott SD. Clopidogrel response variability and future therapies: clopidogrel: does one size fit all? Circulation. 2006;114(22):e600–6.

19. Fefer P, Hod H, Matetzky S. Clopidogrel resistance–the cardiologist's perspective. Platelets. 2007;18(3):175–81.

20. Shuldiner AR, O'Connell JR, Bliden KP, Gandhi A, Ryan K, Horenstein RB, et al. Association of cytochrome P450 2C19 genotype with the antiplatelet effect and clinical efficacy of clopidogrel therapy. JAMA. 2009;302(8):849–57.

21. Storey RF, Husted S, Harrington RA, Heptinstall S, Wilcox RG, Peters G, et al. Inhibition of platelet aggregation by AZD6140, a reversible oral $P2Y_{12}$ receptor antagonist, compared with clopidogrel in patients with acute coronary syndromes. J Am Coll Cardiol. 2007;50(19):1852–6.

22. Wallentin L, Varenhorst C, James S, Erlinge D, Braun OO, Jakubowski JA, et al. Prasugrel achieves greater and faster $P2Y_{12}$ receptor-mediated platelet inhibition than clopidogrel due to more efficient generation of its active metabolite in aspirin-treated patients with coronary artery disease. Eur Heart J. 2008;29(1):21–30.

23. Lip GY, Huber K, Andreotti F, Arnesen H, Airaksinen JK, Cuisset T, et al. Antithrombotic management of atrial fibrillation patients presenting with acute coronary syndrome and/or undergoing coronary stenting: executive summary–a Consensus Document of the European Society of Cardiology Working Group on Thrombosis, endorsed by the European Heart Rhythm Association (EHRA) and the European Association of Percutaneous Cardiovascular Interventions (EAPCI). Eur Heart J. 2010;31(11):1311–8.

24. Ong AT, McFadden EP, Regar E, de Jaegere PP, van Domburg RT, Serruys PW. Late angiographic stent thrombosis (LAST) events with drug-eluting stents. J Am Coll Cardiol. 2005;45(12):2088–92.

25. Stone GW, Moses JW, Ellis SG, Schofer J, Dawkins KD, Morice MC, et al. Safety and efficacy of sirolimus- and paclitaxel-eluting coronary stents. N Engl J Med. 2007;356(10):998–1008.

26. Pfisterer M, Brunner-La Rocca HP, Buser PT, Rickenbacher P, Hunziker P, Mueller C, et al. Late clinical events after clopidogrel discontinuation may limit the benefit of drug-eluting stents: an observational study of drug-eluting versus bare-metal stents. J Am Coll Cardiol. 2006;48(12):2584–91.

27. Park DW, Park S-W, Park K-H, Lee B-K, Kim Y-H, Lee CW, Hong M-K, Kim J-J, Park S-J. Frequency of and risk factors for stent thrombosis after drug-eluting stent implantation during long-term follow-up. Am J Cardiol. 2006;98:352–6.

28. Valgimigli M, Campo G, Percoco G, Monti M, Ferrari F, Tumscitz C, et al. Randomized comparison of 6- versus 24-month clopidogrel therapy after balancing anti-intimal hyperplasia stent potency in all-comer patients undergoing percutaneous coronary intervention Design and rationale for the PROlonging Dual-antiplatelet treatment after Grading stent-induced Intimal hyperplasia study (PRODIGY). Am Heart J. 2010;160(5):804–11.

29. Park SJ, Park DW, Kim YH, Kang SJ, Lee SW, Lee CW, et al. Duration of dual antiplatelet therapy after implantation of drug-eluting stents. Eur Heart J. 2010;362(15):1374–82.

30. Eisenstein EL, Anstrom KJ, Kong DF, Shaw LK, Tuttle RH, Mark DB, et al. Clopidogrel use and long-term clinical outcomes after drug-eluting stent implantation. Jama. 2007;297(2):159–68.

31. Connolly S, Pogue J, Hart R, Pfeffer M, Hohnloser S, Chrolavicius S, et al. Clopidogrel plus aspirin versus oral anticoagulation for atrial fibrillation in the Atrial fibrillation Clopidogrel Trial with Irbesartan for prevention of Vascular Events (ACTIVE W): a randomised controlled trial. Lancet. 2006;367(9526):1903–12.

32. Hart RG, Pearce LA, Aguilar MI. Meta-analysis: antithrombotic therapy to prevent stroke in patients who have nonvalvular atrial fibrillation. Ann Intern Med. 2007;146(12):857–67.

33. Acar J, Iung B, Boissel JP, Samama MM, Michel PL, Teppe JP, et al. AREVA: multicenter randomized comparison of low-dose versus standard-dose anticoagulation in patients with mechanical prosthetic heart valves. Circulation. 1996;94(9):2107–12.

34. Cannegieter SC, Rosendaal FR, Wintzen AR, van der Meer FJ, Vandenbroucke JP, Briet E. Optimal oral anticoagulant therapy in patients with mechanical heart valves. N Engl J Med. 1995;333(1):11–7.

35. Bauersachs R, Berkowitz SD, Brenner B, Buller HR, Decousus H, Gallus AS, et al. Oral rivaroxaban for symptomatic venous thromboembolism. N Engl J Med. 2010;363(26):2499–510.

36. Lagerstedt CI, Olsson CG, Fagher BO, Oqvist BW, Albrechtsson U. Need for long-term anticoagulant treatment in symptomatic calf-vein thrombosis. Lancet. 1985;2(8454):515–8.

37. Schulman S, Granqvist S, Holmstrom M, Carlsson A, Lindmarker P, Nicol P, et al. The duration of oral anticoagulant therapy after a second episode of venous thromboembolism. The Duration of Anticoagulation Trial Study Group. N Engl J Med. 1997; 336(6):393–8.

38. Kearon C, Ginsberg JS, Kovacs MJ, Anderson DR, Wells P, Julian JA, et al. Comparison of low-intensity warfarin therapy with conventional-intensity warfarin therapy for long-term prevention of recurrent venous thromboembolism. N Engl J Med. 2003;349(7):631–9.

39. Doukctis JD. Combination warfarin-ASA therapy: which patients should receive it, which patients should not, and why? Thrombo Res. 2011;127(6):513–7.

40. Buresly K, Eisenberg MJ, Zhang X, Pilote L. Bleeding complications associated with combinations of aspirin, thienopyridine derivatives, and warfarin in elderly patients following acute myocardial infarction. Arch Intern Med. 2005;165(7):784–9.

41. Hurlen M, Abdelnoor M, Smith P, Erikssen J, Arnesen H. Warfarin, aspirin, or both after myocardial infarction. N Engl J Med. 2002;347(13):969–74.

42. Lamberts M, Olesen JB, Ruwald MH, Hansen CM, Karasoy D, Kristensen SL, et al. Bleeding after initiation of multiple antithrombotic drugs, including triple therapy, in atrial fibrillation patients following myocardial infarction and coronary intervention: a nationwide cohort study. Circulation. 2012;126(10):1185–93.

43. Nguyen MC, Lim YL, Walton A, Lefkovits J, Agnelli G, Goodman SG, et al. Combining warfarin and antiplatelet therapy after coronary stenting in the Global Registry of Acute Coronary Events: is it safe and effective to use just one antiplatelet agent? Eur Heart J. 2007;28(14):1717–22.

44. Van de Werf F, Bax J, Betriu A, Blomstrom-Lundqvist C, Crea F, Falk V, et al. Management of acute myocardial infarction in patients presenting with persistent ST-segment elevation: the Task Force on the Management of ST-Segment Elevation Acute Myocardial Infarction of the European Society of Cardiology. Eur Heart J. 2008; 29(23):2909–45.

45. Fuster V, Ryden LE, Cannom DS, Crijns HJ, Curtis AB, Ellenbogen KA, et al. ACC/AHA/ESC 2006 Guidelines for the Management of Patients with Atrial Fibrillation: a report of the American College of Cardiology/American Heart Association Task Force on Practice Guidelines and the European Society of Cardiology Committee for Practice Guidelines (Writing Committee to Revise the 2001 Guidelines for the Management of Patients With Atrial Fibrillation): developed in collaboration with the European Heart Rhythm Association and the Heart Rhythm Society. Circulation. 2006;114(7): e257–354.

46. Hansen ML, Sorensen R, Clausen MT, Fog-Petersen ML, Raunso J, Gadsboll N, et al. Risk of bleeding with single, dual, or triple therapy with warfarin, aspirin, and clopidogrel in patients with atrial fibrillation. Arch Intern Med. 2010;170(16):1433–41.

47. Alexander JH, Lopes RD, James S, Kilaru R, He Y, Mohan P, et al. Apixaban with antiplatelet therapy after acute coronary syndrome. N Engl J Med. 2011;365(8):699–708.

48. Oldgren J, Budaj A, Granger CB, Khder Y, Roberts J, Siegbahn A, et al. Dabigatran vs. placebo in patients with acute coronary syndromes on dual antiplatelet therapy: a randomized, double-blind, phase II trial. Eur Heart J. 2011;32(22):2781–9.

49. Mega JL, Braunwald E, Wiviott SD, Bassand JP, Bhatt DL, Bode C, et al. Rivaroxaban in patients with a recent acute coronary syndrome. N Engl J Med. 2012;366(1):9–19.

50. Mega JL, Braunwald E, Mohanavelu S, Burton P, Poulter R, Misselwitz F, et al. Rivaroxaban versus placebo in patients with acute coronary syndromes (ATLAS ACS-TIMI 46): a randomised, double-blind, phase II trial. Lancet. 2009;374(9683):29–38.

51. Dans AL, Connolly SJ, Wallentin L, Yang S, Nakamya J, Brueckmann M, et al. Concomitant use of antiplatelet therapy with dabigatran or warfarin in the randomized evaluation of long-term anticoagulation therapy (RE-LY) trial. Circulation. 2013;127(5):634–40.

52. Lip GY, Huber K, Andreotti F, Arnesen H, Airaksinen KJ, Cuisset T, et al. Management of antithrombotic therapy in atrial fibrillation patients presenting with acute coronary syndrome and/or

undergoing percutaneous coronary intervention/stenting. Thromb Haemost. 2010;103(1):13–28.

53. Camm AJ, Lip GY, De Caterina R, Savelieva I, Atar D, Hohnloser SH, et al. 2012 focused update of the ESC Guidelines for the management of atrial fibrillation: an update of the 2010 ESC Guidelines for the management of atrial fibrillation. Developed with the special contribution of the European Heart Rhythm Association. Eur Heart J. 2012;33(21):2719–47.

54. Pisters R, Lane DA, Nieuwlaat R, de Vos CB, Crijns HJ, Lip GY. A novel user-friendly score (HAS-BLED) to assess 1-year risk of major bleeding in patients with atrial fibrillation: the Euro Heart Survey. Chest. 2010;138(5):1093–100.

55. Gage BF, Yan Y, Milligan PE, Waterman AD, Culverhouse R, Rich MW, et al. Clinical classification schemes for predicting hemorrhage: results from the National Registry of Atrial Fibrillation (NRAF). Am Heart J. 2006;151(3):713–9.

56. Fang MC, Go AS, Chang Y, Borowsky LH, Pomernacki NK, Udaltsova N, et al. A new risk scheme to predict warfarin-associated hemorrhage: the ATRIA (Anticoagulation and Risk Factors in Atrial Fibrillation) Study. J Am Coll Cardiol. 2011;58(4):395–401.

57. Subherwal S, Bach RG, Chen AY, Gage BF, Rao SV, Newby LK, et al. Baseline risk of major bleeding in non-ST-segment-elevation myocardial infarction: the CRUSADE (Can Rapid risk stratification of Unstable angina patients Suppress ADverse outcomes with Early implementation of the ACC/AHA Guidelines) Bleeding Score. Circulation. 2009;119(14):1873–82.

58. Moscucci M, Fox KA, Cannon CP, Klein W, Lopez-Sendon J, Montalescot G, et al. Predictors of major bleeding in acute coronary syndromes: the Global Registry of Acute Coronary Events (GRACE). Eur Heart J. 2003;24(20):1815–23.

59. Olesen JB, Lip GY, Hansen PR, Lindhardsen J, Ahlehoff O, Andersson C, et al. Bleeding risk in 'real world' patients with atrial fibrillation: comparison of two established bleeding prediction schemes in a nationwide cohort. J Thromb Haemost. 2011;9(8): 1460–7.

60. Apostolakis S, Lane DA, Guo Y, Buller H, Lip GY. Performance of the HEMORR 2 HAGES, ATRIA, and HAS-BLED bleeding risk-prediction scores in nonwarfarin anticoagulated atrial fibrillation patients. J Am Coll Cardiol. 2013;61(3):386–7.

61. Amador P, Santos JF, Goncalves S, Seixo F, Soares L. Comparison of ischemic and bleeding risk scores in non-ST elevation acute coronary syndromes. Acute Card Care. 2011;13(2):68–75.

62. Ho PM, Maddox TM, Wang L, Fihn SD, Jesse RL, Peterson ED, et al. Risk of adverse outcomes associated with concomitant use of clopidogrel and proton pump inhibitors following acute coronary syndrome. JAMA. 2009;301(9):937–44.

63. O'Donoghue ML, Braunwald E, Antman EM, Murphy SA, Bates ER, Rozenman Y, et al. Pharmacodynamic effect and clinical efficacy of clopidogrel and prasugrel with or without a proton-pump inhibitor: an analysis of two randomised trials. Lancet. 2009;374(9694):989–97.
64. Charlot M, Ahlehoff O, Norgaard ML, Jorgensen CH, Sorensen R, Abildstrom SZ, et al. Proton-pump inhibitors are associated with increased cardiovascular risk independent of clopidogrel use: a nationwide cohort study. Ann Intern Med. 2010;153(6):378–86.
65. Bhatt DL, Cryer BL, Contant CF, Cohen M, Lanas A, Schnitzer TJ, et al. Clopidogrel with or without omeprazole in coronary artery disease. N Engl J Med. 2010;363(20):1909–17.
66. Abraham NS, Hlatky MA, Antman EM, Bhatt DL, Bjorkman DJ, Clark CB, et al. ACCF/ACG/AHA 2010 Expert Consensus Document on the concomitant use of proton pump inhibitors and thienopyridines: a focused update of the ACCF/ACG/AHA 2008 expert consensus document on reducing the gastrointestinal risks of antiplatelet therapy and NSAID use: a report of the American College of Cardiology Foundation Task Force on Expert Consensus Documents. Circulation. 2010;122(24):2619–33.
67. Hallas J, Dall M, Andries A, Andersen BS, Aalykke C, Hansen JM, et al. Use of single and combined antithrombotic therapy and risk of serious upper gastrointestinal bleeding: population based case–control study. BMJ. 2006;333(7571):726.
68. Sarafoff N, Ndrepepa G, Mehilli J, Dorrler K, Schulz S, Iijima R, et al. Aspirin and clopidogrel with or without phenprocoumon after drug eluting coronary stent placement in patients on chronic oral anticoagulation. J Intern Med. 2008;264(5):472–80.
69. Rossini R, Musumeci G, Lettieri C, Molfese M, Mihalcsik L, Mantovani P, et al. Long-term outcomes in patients undergoing coronary stenting on dual oral antiplatelet treatment requiring oral anticoagulant therapy. Am J Cardiol. 2008;102(12):1618–23.

Chapter 7
Management of Bleeding Complications

Marcel Levi

Introduction

Anticoagulant agents are often used for prevention and treatment of a wide range of cardiovascular diseases, including acute coronary syndromes. The most frequently used anticoagulants are heparin or its derivatives, vitamin K antagonists (such as warfarin or coumadin) and antiplatelet agents, including aspirin and thienopyridine derivatives, such as clopidogrel or prasugrel. A myriad of clinical studies have demonstrated that these agents (alone or in combination) can prevent or treat acute or chronic thrombo-embolic complications, such as in patients with atrial fibrillation or prosthetic heart valves, after myocardial infarction, percutaneous coronary interventions, or ischemic stroke, and in patients with venous thrombosis or pulmonary embolism [1]. The most important complication of treatment with anticoagulants is hemorrhage, which may be serious, may cause

M. Levi, MD, PhD (✉)
Department of Medicine,
Academic Medical Center,
University of Amsterdam,
Meibergdreef 9, Amsterdam, 1105 AZ,
The Netherlands
e-mail: m.m.levi@amc.uva.nl

P. Avanzas, P. Clemmensen (eds.), *Pharmacological Treatment*   213
of Acute Coronary Syndromes, Current Cardiovascular Therapy,
DOI 10.1007/978-1-4471-5424-2_7,
© Springer-Verlag London 2014

long-term debilitating disease, or may even be life-threatening [2, 3]. In a very large series of 34,146 patients with acute ischemic coronary syndromes, anticoagulant-associated bleeding was associated with a 5-fold increased risk of death during the first 30 days and a 1.5-fold higher mortality between 30 days and 6 months [4]. Major bleeding was an independent predictor of mortality across all subgroups that were analyzed. In some clinical situations the incidence of serious bleeding complications may annihilate or even overwhelm the efficacy of antithrombotic agents, as has been shown in the secondary prevention of patients with ischemic stroke by vitamin K antagonists [5]. Nevertheless, in many situations clinical studies show a favorable balance between efficacy and safety in favor of anticoagulant treatment. However, if severe bleeding occurs or if a patient needs to undergo an urgent invasive procedure, such as emergency surgery, it may be necessary to reverse the anticoagulant effect of the various agents [6]. Depending on the clinical situation, i.e. the severity of the bleeding or the urgency and estimated risk of the invasive procedure, this reversal may take place in a few hours, but in some cases immediate reversal is necessary (Table 7.1) [7, 8]. Generally, each (immediate) reversal of anticoagulant treatment needs also to take into consideration the indication for the antithrombotic agents. For example, the interruption of combined aspirin and clopidogrel treatment in a patient in whom recently an intracoronary stent has been inserted will markedly increase the risk of acute stent thrombosis with consequent downstream cardiac ischemia or infarction. Likewise, in a patient with a prosthetic mitral valve and atrial fibrillation, interruption of vitamin K antagonists may increase the risk of valve thrombosis and cerebral or systemic embolism. Each of these specific clinical situations requires a careful and balanced assessment of the benefits and risks of reversing anticoagulants (and potential strategies to keep the period of reversal as short as possible). In this chapter, we will describe the various strategies to reverse the anticoagulant effect of currently most widely used antithrombotic agents and the new generation of anticoagulants.

TABLE 7.1 Reversal of anticoagulant effect of different agents

	Time until restoration of hemostasis after cessation of therapeutic dose	Antidote	Remark
Heparin	3–4 h	Protamine sulphate 25–30 mg; immediate reversal	1 mg of protamin per 100 anti-Xa units given in the last 2–3 h
LMW heparin	12–24 h	(Partially) protamine sulphate 25–50 mg; immediate reversal	1 mg of protamine per 100 anti-Xa units given in the last 8 h
Pentasaccharides	Fondaparinux: 24–30 h Idraparinux: 5–15 days	Recombinant factor VIIa 90 ug/kg; immediate thrombin generation	Based on laboratory end-points, no systematic experience in bleeding patients
Vitamin K antagonists	Acenocoumarol: 18–24 h Warfarin: 60–80 h Phenprocoumon: 8–10 days	Vitamin K i.v: reversal in 12–16 h Vitamin K orally: reversal in 24 h PCC's: immediate reversal	Dose of vitamin K or PCC's depend of INR and bodyweight
Oral thrombin and factor Xa inhibitors	Dependent of compound, usually within 12 h	Prothrombin complex concentrates or recombinant factor Xa for Xa inhibitors, unsure for IIa inhibitors	Based on laboratory end-points, no systematic experience in bleeding patients

(continued)

TABLE 7.1 (continued)

	Time until restoration of hemostasis after cessation of therapeutic dose	Antidote	Remark
Aspirin	5–10 days (time to produce unaffected platelets)	DDAVP (0.3–0.4 ug/kg) and/or platelet concentrate; reversal in 15–30 min	Cessation not always required, also dependent on clinical situation and indication
Clopidogrel Prasugrel	1–2 days	Platelet concentrate, possibly in combination with DDAVP (0.3–0.4 ug/kg); reversal in 15–30 min	Cessation not always desirable, also dependent on clinical situation and indication

LMW heparin low molecular weight heparin, *PCC* prothrombin complex concentrate, *DDAVP* de-amino d-arginin vasopressin or desmo pressin

Incidence and Risk Factors for Bleeding in Patients on Anticoagulants

In well-controlled patients in clinical trials treatment with heparin or vitamin K antagonists (VKA's) increase the risk of major bleeding by 0.5 %/year and the risk of intracranial hemorrhage by about 0.2 %/year [9]. The most important risk factor for hemorrhage in users of anticoagulants is the intensity of the anticoagulant effect [9]. Studies indicate that with a target INR of >3.0 the incidence of major bleeding is twice as large as in studies with a target INR of 2.0–3.0 [10]. In a meta-analysis of studies in patients with prosthetic heart valves, a lower INR target range resulted in a lower frequency of major bleeding and intracranial hemorrhage with a similar anti-thrombotic efficacy [11]. A retrospective analysis of outpatients using warfarin who presented with intracranial hemorrhage demonstrated that the risk of this complication doubled for each 1 unit increment of the INR [12]. Patient characteristics constitute another important determinant of the bleeding risk bleeding. Elderly patients have a 2-fold increased risk of bleeding [13] and the relative risk of intracranial hemorage (in particular at higher intensities of anticoagulation) was 2.5 (95 % CI 2.3–9.4) in patients >85 years compared to patients 70–74 year old [14]. Recently, genetic factors have been identified that may affect the risk of bleeding. Common polymorphisms in the P450 CYP2C9 enzyme were found to be associated with slow metabolism of VKA's and (possibly) a higher risk of bleeding [9, 15]. Other genetic factors that may influence the requirement of VKA's are variants in the vitamin K epoxide reductase complex subunit 1 gene (*VKORC1*) [16]. Co-morbidity, such as renal or hepatic insufficiency, may also significantly increase the risk of bleeding. A case-control study in 1,986 patients on VKA's showed that this comorbidity increased the risk of bleeding by about 2.5 [17]. Another very important determinant of the risk of bleeding is the use of other medication, in particular agents affecting platelet function. Two meta-analyses, comprising 6 trials with a total of 3,874 patients and 10 trials with a total of

5,938 patients, found a relative risk of major bleeding when VKA's or heparin were combined with aspirin of 2.4 (95 % CI 1.2–4.8) and 2.5 (95 % CI 1.7–3.7), respectively [18, 19]. A population-based case-control study confirmed the high risk of upper gastro-intestinal bleeding in patients using VKA's in combination with aspirin and/or clopidogrel [20]. Non-steroidal anti-inflammatory agents (NSAIDs) are also associated with an enhanced risk of gastro-intestinal bleeding. The combined use of VKA's and NSAIDs may result in an 11-fold higher risk of hospitalization for gastro-intestinal bleeding as compared to the general population [21]. This risk is not significantly lower when using selective inhibitors of COX-2 [22].

Heparin and Low Molecular Weight (LMW) Heparin

Heparin and heparin derivatives act by binding to antithrombin and thereby about 1,000-fold potentiating the anticoagulant effect of this endogenous inhibitor towards thrombin and factor Xa (and some other coagulation factors). Heparin has a relatively short half life of about 60–90 min and therefore the anticoagulant effect of therapeutic doses of heparin will be mostly eliminated at 3–4 h after termination of continuous intravenous administration [23]. The anticoagulant effect of high dose subcutaneous heparin, however, will take a longer time to abolish. If a more immediate neutralization of heparin is required, intravenous protamine sulphate is the antidote of choice. Protamine, derived from fish sperm, binds to heparin to from a stable biologically inactive complex. Each mg of protamine will neutralize approximately 100 units of heparin. Hence, the protamine dose in a patient on a stable therapeutic heparin dose of 1,000–1,250 U/h should be about 25–30 mg (sufficient to block the amount of heparin given in the last 2–3 h). The maximum dose of protamine is 50 mg. Since the half-life of protamine is only about 10 min, the reversal of therapeutic dose subcutaneous heparin requires a repeated infusion of protamine sulphate (e.g. repeated after 1 h). The effect of protamine can be monitored by measuring the activated partial thromboplastin time (aPTT), which should normalize after its administration.

The reversal of LMW heparin is more complex, as protamine sulphate will only neutralize the anti-factor IIa activity and has no or only partial effect on the smaller heparin fragments causing the anti-factor Xa activity of the compound [24, 25]. The net effect of protamine reversal of LMW heparin is not completely clear. There are no clinical studies that have systematically studied this and small case series and experimental animal studies show contradictory results [25–27]. As the aPTT is not useful as a monitoring assay when using LMW heparin, it can also not be used for the monitoring of the neutralizing effect of protamine. Given the relatively long half-life of LMW heparin, the lack of an adequate strategy to reverse its anticoagulant action may sometimes cause a problem in clinical situations. A practical approach is to give 1 mg of protamine per 100 anti-factor Xa units of LMW heparin given in the last 8 h (whereas 1 mg of enoxaparin equals 100 anti-factor Xa units). If bleeding continues, a second dose of 0.5 mg per 100 anti-factor Xa units can be given.

The most important adverse effect of protamine is an allergic response, including hemodynamic and respiratory problems [28]. Most adverse reactions can be prevented or minimized by slowing the rate of administration of the drug or by pretreatment with steroids and antihistamines. Risk factors for an adverse reaction are sensitivity to fish (as may occur in traditional fishermen that are often exposed to fish proteins when cutting themselves), a history of vasectomy (which may demolish the blood-testis barrier with consequent formation of anti-semen antibodies) and a history of receiving protamine sulphate containing insulin. Initial reports that the use of protamine sulphate could lead to an increased risk of rebound thrombosis, in particular ischemic stroke [29, 30], were not confirmed in a recent randomized controlled study [31].

There are some other strategies to reverse (mostly unfractionated) heparin, such as platelet factor-4, heparanase, or extracorporeal heparin-removal devices, but none of these approaches have been properly evaluated and they are not currently approved for clinical use [32–34].

Pentasaccharides

Pentasaccharides are recently developed synthetic compounds that effectively bind and potentiate antithrombin to block factor Xa. Since they lack the additional glycosaminoglycan saccharide residues to bind to thrombin, it has an effect on factor Xa exclusively. The prototype pentasaccharide (and the only one approved for clinical use so far) is fondaparinux. Another pentasaccharide that is currently under study is idraparinux. The main difference between these two agents is the elimination half-life, which is 15–20 h for fondaparinux and 5½ days for idraparinux. This means that idraparinux can be administered once weekly, which renders the subcutaneous route of administration less cumbersome. Pentasaccharides were shown to be effective in the prophylaxis and treatment of venous thromboembolism and are currently evaluated in other types of thrombosis [35]. The (very) long half-life of pentasaccharides necessitates the availability of a suitable antidote if major bleeding complicates the treatment, which may especially occur in patients that are treated with therapeutic doses of this type of anticoagulation. So far, there is no antidote for pentasaccharides that has been studied in controlled clinical studies [36]. The only agent that has been systematically evaluated to reverse the anticoagulant effect of pentasaccharides is recombinant factor VIIa (rVIIa). Two randomized placebo-controlled studies in healthy volunteers have tested the hypothesis that rVIIa may be useful as a suitable antidote for pentasaccharide anticoagulation [37, 38]. In the first study 16 subjects were treated with therapeutic doses of the pentasaccharide fondaparinux and after 2 h (at the time of maximal anticoagulation) challenged with rVIIa or placebo. Injection of rVIIa (90 μg/kg) after fondaparinux normalized the prolonged aPTT and prothrombin time (PT) and reversed the decrease in prothrombin activation fragments $1+2$ $(F(1+2))$, as observed with fondaparinux alone. Thrombin-generation time and endogenous thrombin potential, which were inhibited by fondaparinux, normalized up to 6 h after rVIIa injection. In the second study 12 subjects received a single s.c. dose of 7.5 mg idraparinux (which is 3 fold higher than the currently recommended dose). The inhibition of thrombin generation by idraparinux, as reflected by an increased thrombin generation time (TGT) and decreased level of prothrombin fragment $1+2$ (F_{1+2}), was partially reversed by injection of rVIIa 3 h after idraparinux administration. The administration of rVIIa 1 week after treatment with idraparinux (when much lower, though still therapeutic, doses of the pentasaccharide were present) resulted in an nearly complete reversal of anticoagulation, reflected by normalization of thrombin generation time and other markers of thrombin generation. As mentioned, there are no controlled trials in patients who present with pentasaccharide-induced bleeding but there is some anecdotal experience suggesting that rVIIa may indeed be able to stop bleeding in patients anticoagulated with fondaparinux.

Vitamin K Antagonists

When interrupting the administration of VKA's important differences in the half-lives of the various agents (9 h for acenocoumarol, 36–42 h for warfarin, and 90 h for phenprocoumon, respectively) need to be taken into account [39]. The most straightforward intervention to counteract the effect of VKA's is the administration of vitamin K [40]. There is quite some debate on the use of vitamin K in patients with a too high INR but no signs of bleeding. However, a recent randomized controlled trial did not find any difference in bleeding or other complications in nonbleeding patients with INR values of 4.5 to 10 that were treated with vitamin K or placebo [41]. In patients with clinically significant bleeding administration of vitamin K is crucial to reverse the anticoagulant effect of VKA's. Vitamin K can be given orally and intravenously, whereas the parenteral route has the advantage of a more rapid onset of the treatment [42]. After the administration of i.v. vitamin K, within 2 h the INR will start to drop and will be completely normalized within 12–16 h [43], whereas after oral administration it will take up to 24 h to normalize the INR [40]. Intramuscular injections of vitamin K should be avoided in patients who are anticoagulated and subcutaneous administration of vitamin K results in a less predictable bioavailability [42]. A potential concern with the use of parenteral vitamin K is the occurrence of anaphylactic reactions, although the incidence of this complication is very low, in particular with the more modern micelle preparations [44].

In case of very serious or even life-threatening bleeding, immediate correction of the INR is mandatory and can be achieved by the administration of vitamin K-dependent coagulation factors. Theoretically, these factors are present in fresh frozen plasma, however, the amount of plasma that is required to correct the INR is very large, carries the risk of fluid overload, and will probably take hours to administer [45]. Therefore, prothrombin complex concentrates (PCC's), containing all vitamin K-dependent coagulation factors, are more useful. Although PCC's can indeed be given using fixed dose schemes, it has been shown that individualized dosing regimens based on INR at presentation and body weight are more effective [46]. In a prospective study in patients using VKA and presenting with bleeding also found that PCC's resulted in at least satisfactory and sustained hemostasis in 98 % [47]. In recent years the safety of PCC's, in particular regarding the transmission of blood-borne infectious diseases, has markedly improved owing to several techniques, such as pasteurization, nanofiltration, and addition of solvent detergent. The risk of disseminated intravascular coagulation (DIC) due to traces of activated coagulation factors in PCC's comes from older literature and modern PCC's seem not to be associated with eliciting DIC [48].

New Direct Factor Xa Inhibitors

In recent years a large number of new antithrombotic agents has been developed and tested in clinical trials and many of these new agents will become available for clinical practice in the very near future [49]. The need for new anticoagulant agents is quite obvious; Firstly, the current agents are insufficiently effective. For example 10–15 % of patients undergoing major orthopedic surgery develop venous thromboembolism, despite prophylaxis with low molecular weight (LMW) heparin [50]. Furthermore, the available anticoagulants are relatively unsafe, mostly due to the occurrence of bleeding as discussed hereabove. Lastly, current anticoagulant agents are often cumbersome with regards to their clinical use, requiring repeated laboratory control and frequent dose adjustments. Increasing knowledge on the function of the haemostatic system *in vivo* has resulted in a new generation of anticoagulant agents.

Some of these new class of anticoagulants are directed at factor Xa. Prototypes of these agents are rivaroxaban and apixaban, which have shown promising results in clinical studies [51, 52]. In trials in patients with acute venous thromboembolism rivaroxaban and apixaban were as effective as LMW heparin but rivaroxaban was associated with a lower incidence of bleeding complications (2.2 % versus 8.8 %) [53, 54]. Rivaroxaban was also studied in patients with acute coronary syndromes and showed a dose-dependent efficacy but also increased rates of major bleeding at higher doses [55]. Similarly, apixaban showed a similar pattern and exhibited 2.5 fold increased bleeding rates, in particular in patients using simultaneous anti-platelet agents [56]. Taken together, compared to LMW heparin direct factor Xa inhibitors result at doses achieving equivalent efficacy a lower bleeding risk and at doses achieving higher efficacy a similar bleeding risk. This means that for some clinical situations these drugs may represent an important improvement, however, the risk of (major) bleeding is still present. Recently it was shown that the administration of prothrombin complex concentrate

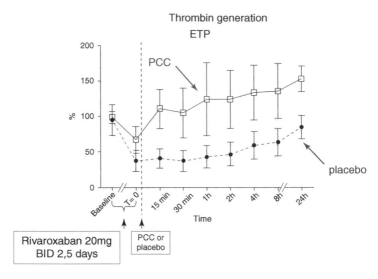

FIGURE 7.1 Restoration of rivaroxaban-induced impaired thrombin generation, measured by endogenous thrombin potential (*ETP*), by administration of prothrombin complex concentrates (*squares*) as compared to placebo (*circles*) in healthy volunteers. Mean ± SD are reported, the difference between the two groups is statistically significant (p < 0.001 Repeated Measures ANOVA)

(PCC) resulted in a correction of the prolonged prothrombin time and restored depressed thrombin generation after rivaroxaban treatment in a controlled trial in healthy human subjects (Fig. 7.1) [57]. The effect of PCC's on reversal of the anticoagulant effect of oral factor Xa inhibitors was confirmed in a series of experiments in animals and human subjects [58–60]. The clinical efficacy in bleeding patients, however, needs to be established.

Direct Thrombin Inhibitors

Another important group of new anticoagulants is the class of direct thrombin inhibitors. Thrombin is the central enzyme in the coagulation process, not only mediating the conversion of fibrinogen to fibrin, but also being the most important physiological activator of platelets and various other coagulation factors. Inhibition of thrombin can be achieved by administration of heparin, but in view of the limited capability of the heparin-antithrombin complex to inhibit surface-bound thrombin, new antithrombin-independent anticoagulants have been developed [61]. Prototype of these thrombin inhibitors is hirudin, originally derived from the saliva from leeches (*hirudo medicinalis*) and nowadays produced by recombinant technology. Melagatran is a synthetic thrombin inhibitor, which has predictable pharmacokinetic properties and can thus be used in a fixed dose [62]. Moreover, the pro-drug ximelagatran is relatively quickly absorbed after oral ingestion and results in a sufficient systemic availability, rendering this agent suitable for long-term use as oral anticoagulant. Despite clinical trials on prevention and treatment of venous thromboembolism and in patients with atrial fibrillation showing a promising efficacy of ximelagatran, the compound has been withdrawn by the manufacturer, due to the occurrence of enhanced liver enzymes in 6–7 % of patients. Recently, dabigatran, also a direct thrombin inhibitor with good and relatively stable bioavailability after oral ingestion, has been introduced and licensed for prevention of venous thromboembolism after orthopedic surgery. Indeed, clinical trials evaluating dabigatran against LMW heparin in patients undergoing major othropedic surgery show similar or slightly better efficacy of the direct thrombin inhibtor and similar bleeding rates [63, 64]. The largest group of patients using long-term anticoagulants, however, are those with atrial fibrillation. In these patients dabigatran (150 mg twice daily) showed a significantly lower rate of thromboembolic complications compared to warfarin (relative risk 0.66; 95 % confidence interval 0.53–0.82) but also a slightly lower risk of major hemorrhage (3.11 %/year in the dabigatran group versus 3.36 %/year in the warfarin group) [65]. Based on these findings and if confirmed by other ongoing major trials, it may be quite likely that in the future oral anticoagulant treatment with vitamin K antagonists is going to be replaced by treatment with directly acting anti-coagulants, such as direct thrombin inhibitors. However, the risk of major bleeding is still relatively large and requires adequate management strategies.

For each of the direct thrombin inhibitors no established antidote is available in case of serious bleeding complicating the anticoagulant treatment. Again, the half-life of most of the agents is relatively short, hence in case of less serious bleeding interruption of treatment will be sufficient to reverse the anticoagulant effect. However, if immediate reversal is required, it is not clear which would be the best strategy. In a controlled clinical study in healthy subjects the melagatran-induced effects on aPTT, thrombin generation and platelet activation were not affected by the administration of rVIIa [66]. Also, in human subjects challenged with dabigatran there was no reversal of the anticoagulation by administration of prothrombin complex concentrates [57]. An experimental study of intracerebral hematoma in dabigatran-treated rats, however, demonstrated that relatively high doses of prothrombin complex concentrates were able to reduce hematoma volume [67].

Aspirin

Aspirin is effective in the secondary prevention of athero-thrombotic disease, in particular coronary artery disease, cerebrovascular thromboembolism and peripheral arterial disease [68]. As a consequence, aspirin is one of the most widely used agents in the Western world. Aspirin increases the risk of bleeding, in particular gastro-intestinal bleeding, and has been associated with a small but consistent increase in intracerebral hemorrhage. In addition, it has been shown that the use of aspirin is associated with increased perioperative blood loss in major procedures, although this does not necessarily translates into clinically relevant endpoints, such as the requirement for transfusion or re-operation [69]. Over the last years the approach to the patient who uses aspirin and who presents with bleeding or needs to undergo an invasive procedure has changed considerably. In fact, in current clinical practice bleeding can almost always be managed with local hemostatic procedures or conservative strategies without interrupting aspirin and also most invasive procedures do not require the cessation of aspirin when adequate attention is given to local hemostasis. In contrast, interruption of aspirin has been associated with an increased risk of thromboembolic complications, potentially due to a rebound hypercoagulability. Obviously, in special clinical circumstances, such as intracranial bleeding or the need to undergo a neurosurgical or ophthalmic procedure, the anti-hemostatic effect of aspirin needs to be reversed immediately. The most rigorous measure to achieve that is the administration of platelet concentrate after cessation of aspirin. Another approach is the administration of de-amino d-arginin vasopressin (DDAVP, desmopressin). DDAVP is a vasopressin analogue that despite minor molecular differences has retained its antidiuretic properties but has much less vaso-active effects [70]. DDAVP induces release of the contents of the endothelial cell associated Weibel Palade bodies, including von Willebrand factor. Hence, the administration of DDAVP results in a marked increase in the plasma concentration of von Willebrand factor (and associated coagulation factor VIII) and (also by yet unexplained additional mechanisms) a remarkable augmentation of primary hemostasis as a consequence. DDAVP is effective in patients with mild hemophilia A or von Willebrand's disease and in patients with qualitative platelet defects, such as in uremia or liver cirrhosis. DDAVP seems also capable of correcting the aspirin-induced platelet dysfunction, although large clinical studies employing relevant outcome parameters are missing [71]. The combined effect of platelet concentrate and subsequent administration of DDAVP has also been advocated to correct the aspirin effect on platelets. The standard dose of DDAVP is 0.3–0.4 µg/kg in 100 ml saline over 30 min and its effect is immediate.

Thienopyridine Derivatives

Clopidogrel, prasugrel and ticagrelor belong to the class of thienopyridine derivatives, which act by blocking the adenosine diphosphate (ADP) receptor on the platelet. Clinical studies have shown that clopidogrel is as good as aspirin in the secondary prevention of atherothrombotic events [72]. Importantly, the combination of aspirin and clopidogrel is vastly superior over aspirin alone in patients who have received intracoronary stents or in other patients with high risk coronary artery disease. There is ample evidence that dual platelet inhibition of aspirin plus clopidogrel has a significantly higher efficacy than aspirin alone in patients with acute coronary syndromes who have undergone coronary interventions for at least a year (and possibly longer) after the event. However, the increased efficacy of the combined use of aspirin and clopidogrel is also associated with a significantly higher bleeding risk [73]. Prasugrel is another thienopyridine derivative that after rapid and almost complete absorption after oral ingestion irreversibly binds to the ADP receptor. Prasugrel has a stronger anti-platelet effect than clopidogrel because of more effective metabolism and less dependence of cytochrome P450 enzymes that may be subject to genetic polymorphisms [74]. Prasugrel was shown to be more effective than clopidogrel in preventing ischemic events in patients with ST elevation myocardial infarction undergoing primary percutaneous coronary interventions (with or without stent) [75]. Rates of major bleeding were similar between clopidogrel and prasugrel, however, the rate of serious bleeding in patients requiring emergency coronary artery bypass grafting (CABG) was higher in the prasugrel group. In patients with acute coronary syndromes prasugrel was also more effective than clopidogrel in preventing cardiovascular death, myocardial infarction and stroke, however, major bleeding rates were higher in the prasugrel group (2.4 % versus 1.8 %) [76]. Of note, this disadvantage of prasugrel did not outweigh the efficacy benefit, and the net clinical benefit (defined as the efficacy gain minus the increased risk of major bleeding) was preserved in favour of prasugrel. Ticagrelor is a cyclopentyltriazolopyrimidine that differs from thienopyridines (ticlopidin, clopidogrel, prasugrel), as ticagrelor is not a prodrug requiring active biotransformation by cytochromes in the liver and thus is characterized by a more rapid, more effective and more consistent platelet inhibition than ticlopidin or clopidogrel [77]. The Platelet Inhibition and Patient Outcomes (PLATO) trial determined whether ticagrelor was superior to clopidogrel for the prevention of vascular events and death in a broad population of patients presenting with an acute coronary syndrome [78]. treatment with ticagrelor as compared with clopidogrel significantly reduced the rate of death from vascular causes, myocardial infarction, or stroke. The ticagrelor and clopidogrel groups did not differ significantly with regard to the rates of major bleeding as defined in the trial or according to the Thrombolysis in Myocardial Infarction (TIMI) criteria. The two treatment groups did not differ significantly in the rates of CABG-related major bleeding or bleeding requiring transfusion of red cells. However, in the ticagrelor group, there was a higher rate of non-CABG-related major bleeding according to the study criteria and the TIMI criteria. With ticagrelor as compared with clopidogrel, there were more episodes of intracranial bleeding, including fatal intracranial bleeding. However, there were fewer episodes of other types of fatal bleeding in the ticagrelor group. Recently, a fourth thienopyridine derivative has been introduced: cangrelor. The advantage of this compound over the other members of this group is the faster onset of action, which may be critical in acute coronary syndromes. However, two major clinical trials comparing cangrelor with clopidogrel in patients undergoing percutaneous coronary interventions did not show a higher efficacy of cangrelor but did demonstrate a significantly higher risk of bleeding [79, 80]. Taken together, dual platelet inhibition, in particular with clopidogrel or even more outspoken with prasugrel, is highly effective in high risk patients with coronary artery disease but the bleeding risk with dual platelet inhibition is something to take into account and strategies to reverse the antiplatelet effect may be warranted in case of serious bleeding.

The decision whether or not the interrupt or even reverse antithrombotic treatment with dual platelet inhibition in case of serious bleeding or the need to perform an invasive procedure will depend on the specific clinical situation but also on the indication for the antithrombotic treatment (see above). Especially in patients with recent implantation of an intracoronary stent (in the last 6–12 weeks), cardiologists will often not or only reluctantly agree with cessation of treatment [81]. In this period re-endothelization of the stent has not yet occurred and the patient is very vulnerable to acute thrombotic occlusion of the stent. In patients with drug-eluting stents this period may be even longer. If, however, the decision is made to stop and even reverse the treatment with aspirin and clopidogrel, administration of platelet concentrate is probably the best way to correct the hemostatic defect [82]. In addition, DDAVP was shown to correct the defect in platelet aggregation caused by clopidogrel, so this may be another option [83].

Conclusion

Conventional anticoagulant treatment can be reversed by specific interventions when the clinical situation requires immediate correction of hemostasis. For the new generation of anticoagulants, no specific antidotes are available, although some interventions are promising but need further evaluation. Antiplatelet therapy with aspirin, alone or in combination with thienopyridine derivatives, such as clopidogrel and prasugrel, can be reversed but this is often not required and sometimes not desirable in view of the indication for this treatment.

References

1. Hirsh J, Guyatt G, Albers GW, Harrington R, Schunemann HJ. Antithrombotic and thrombolytic therapy: American College of Chest Physicians Evidence-Based Clinical Practice Guidelines (8th Edition). Chest. 2008;133(6 Suppl):110S–2.

2. Mannucci PM, Levi M. Prevention and treatment of major blood loss. N Engl J Med. 2007;356(22):2301–11.

3. Levi MM, Eerenberg E, Lowenberg E, Kamphuisen PW. Bleeding in patients using new anticoagulants or antiplatelet agents: risk factors and management. Neth J Med. 2010;68(2):68–76.

4. Eikelboom JW, Mehta SR, Anand SS, Xie C, Fox KA, Yusuf S. Adverse impact of bleeding on prognosis in patients with acute coronary syndromes. Circulation. 2006;114(8):774–82.

5. Algra A. Medium intensity oral anticoagulants versus aspirin after cerebral ischaemia of arterial origin (ESPRIT): a randomised controlled trial. Lancet Neurol. 2007;6(2):115–24.

6. Lip GY, Andreotti F, Fauchier L, Huber K, Hylek E, Knight E, Lane DA, Levi M, Marin F, Palareti G, Kirchhof P, Collet JP, Rubboli A, Poli D, Camm J. Bleeding risk assessment and management in atrial fibrillation patients: a position document from the European Heart Rhythm Association, endorsed by the European Society of Cardiology Working Group on Thrombosis. Europace. 2011;13(5): 723–46.

7. Levi M. Emergency reversal of antithrombotic treatment. Intern Emerg Med. 2009;4(2):137–45.

8. Levi M, Eerenberg E, Kamphuisen PW. Bleeding risk and reversal strategies for old and new anticoagulants and antiplatelet agents. J Thromb Haemost. 2011;9(9)1705–12.

9. Schulman S, Beyth RJ, Kearon C, Levine MN. Hemorrhagic complications of anticoagulant and thrombolytic treatment: American College of Chest Physicians Evidence-Based Clinical Practice Guidelines (8th Edition). Chest. 2008;133(6 Suppl):257S–98.

10. Saour JN, Sieck JO, Mamo LA, Gallus AS. Trial of different intensities of anticoagulation in patients with prosthetic heart valves. N Engl J Med. 1990;322(7):428–32.

11. Vink R, Kraaijenhagen RA, Hutten BA, van den Brink RB, de Mol BA, Buller HR, Levi M. The optimal intensity of vitamin K antagonists in patients with mechanical heart valves: a meta-analysis. J Am Coll Cardiol. 2003;42(12):2042–8.

12. Hylek EM, Singer DE. Risk factors for intracranial hemorrhage in outpatients taking warfarin. Ann Intern Med. 1994;120(11): 897–902.

13. Hutten BA, Lensing AW, Kraaijenhagen RA, Prins MH. Safety of treatment with oral anticoagulants in the elderly. A systematic review. Drugs Aging. 1999;14(4):303–12.

14. Fang MC, Chang Y, Hylek EM, Rosand J, Greenberg SM, Go AS, Singer DE. Advanced age, anticoagulation intensity, and risk for intracranial hemorrhage among patients taking warfarin for atrial fibrillation. Ann Intern Med. 2004;141(10):745–52.

15. Higashi MK, Veenstra DL, Kondo LM, Wittkowsky AK, Srinouanprachanh SL, Farin FM, Rettie AE. Association between CYP2C9 genetic variants and anticoagulation-related outcomes during warfarin therapy. JAMA. 2002;287(13):1690–8.

16. Reitsma PH, van der Heijden JF, Groot AP, Rosendaal FR, Buller HR. A C1173T dimorphism in the VKORC1 gene determines coumarin sensitivity and bleeding risk. PLoS Med. 2005;2(10):e312.
17. Levi M, Hovingh GK, Cannegieter SC, Vermeulen M, Buller HR, Rosendaal FR. Bleeding in patients receiving vitamin K antagonists who would have been excluded from trials on which the indication for anticoagulation was based. Blood. 2008;111(9):4471–6.
18. Hart RG, Benavente O, Pearce LA. Increased risk of intracranial hemorrhage when aspirin is combined with warfarin: a meta-analysis and hypothesis. Cerebrovasc Dis. 1999;9(4):215–7.
19. Rothberg MB, Celestin C, Fiore LD, Lawler E, Cook JR. Warfarin plus aspirin after myocardial infarction or the acute coronary syndrome: meta-analysis with estimates of risk and benefit. Ann Intern Med. 2005;143(4):241–50.
20. Hallas J, Dall M, Andries A, Andersen BS, Aalykke C, Hansen JM, Andersen M, Lassen AT. Use of single and combined antithrombotic therapy and risk of serious upper gastrointestinal bleeding: population based case-control study. BMJ. 2006;333(7571):726.
21. Mellemkjaer L, Blot WJ, Sorensen HT, Thomassen L, McLaughlin JK, Nielsen GL, Olsen JH. Upper gastrointestinal bleeding among users of NSAIDs: a population-based cohort study in Denmark. Br J Clin Pharmacol. 2002;53(2):173–81.
22. Battistella M, Mamdami MM, Juurlink DN, Rabeneck L, Laupacis A. Risk of upper gastrointestinal hemorrhage in warfarin users treated with nonselective NSAIDs or COX-2 inhibitors. Arch Intern Med. 2005;165(2):189–92.
23. Hirsh J, Bauer KA, Donati MB, Gould M, Samama MM, Weitz JI. Parenteral anticoagulants: American College of Chest Physicians Evidence-Based Clinical Practice Guidelines (8th Edition). Chest. 2008;133(6 Suppl):141S–59.
24. Lindblad B, Borgstrom A, Wakefield TW, Whitehouse Jr WM, Stanley JC. Protamine reversal of anticoagulation achieved with a low molecular weight heparin. The effects on eicosanoids, clotting and complement factors. Thromb Res. 1987;48(1):31–40.
25. Massonnet-Castel S, Pelissier E, Bara L, Terrier E, Abry B, Guibourt P, Swanson J, Jaulmes B, Carpentier A, Samama M. Partial reversal of low molecular weight heparin (PK 10169) anti-Xa activity by protamine sulfate: in vitro and in vivo study during cardiac surgery with extracorporeal circulation. Haemostasis. 1986;16(2):139–46.
26. Van Ryn-McKenna J, Cai L, Ofosu FA, Hirsh J, Buchanan MR. Neutralization of enoxaparine-induced bleeding by protamine sulfate. Thromb Haemost. 1990;63(2):271–4.
27. Bang CJ, Berstad A, Talstad I. Incomplete reversal of enoxaparin-induced bleeding by protamine sulfate. Haemostasis. 1991;21(3):155–60.
28. Caplan SN, Berkman EM. Letter: protamine sulfate and fish allergy. N Engl J Med. 1976;295(3):172.

29. Fearn SJ, Parry AD, Picton AJ, Mortimer AJ, McCollum CN. Should heparin be reversed after carotid endarterectomy? A randomised prospective trial. Eur J Vasc Endovasc Surg. 1997;13(4):394–7.

30. Mauney MC, Buchanan SA, Lawrence WA, Bishop A, Sinclair K, Daniel TM, Tribble CG, Kron IL. Stroke rate is markedly reduced after carotid endarterectomy by avoidance of protamine. J Vasc Surg. 1995;22(3):264–9.

31. Dellagrammaticas D, Lewis SC, Gough MJ. Is heparin reversal with protamine after carotid endarterectomy dangerous? Eur J Vasc Endovasc Surg. 2008;36(1):41–4.

32. D'Ambra M. Restoration of the normal coagulation process: advances in therapies to antagonize heparin. J Cardiovasc Pharmacol. 1996;27 Suppl 1:S58–62.

33. Despotis GJ, Summerfield AL, Joist JH, Goodnough LT, Santoro SA, Zimmermann JJ, Lappas DG. In vitro reversal of heparin effect with heparinase: evaluation with whole blood prothrombin time and activated partial thromboplastin time in cardiac surgical patients. Anesth Analg. 1994;79(4):670–4.

34. Tao W, Deyo DJ, Brunston Jr RL, Vertrees RA, Zwischenberger JB. Extracorporeal heparin adsorption following cardiopulmonary bypass with a heparin removal device–an alternative to protamine. Crit Care Med. 1998;26(6):1096–102.

35. Buller HR. Treatment of symptomatic venous thromboembolism: improving outcomes. Semin Thromb Hemost. 2002;28 Suppl 2:41–8.

36. Crowther MA, Warkentin TE. Bleeding risk and the management of bleeding complications in patients undergoing anticoagulant therapy: focus on new anticoagulant agents. Blood. 2008;111(10): 4871–9.

37. Bijsterveld NR, Vink R, van Aken BE, Fennema H, Peters RJ, Meijers JC, Buller HR, Levi M. Recombinant factor VIIa reverses the anticoagulant effect of the long-acting pentasaccharide idraparinux in healthy volunteers. Br J Haematol. 2004;124:653–8.

38. Bijsterveld NR, Moons AH, Boekholdt SM, van Aken BE, Fennema H, Peters RJ, Meijers JC, Buller HR, Levi M. Ability of recombinant factor VIIa to reverse the anticoagulant effect of the pentasaccharide fondaparinux in healthy volunteers. Circulation. 2002;106(20): 2550–4.

39. Ansell J, Hirsh J, Hylek E, Jacobson A, Crowther M, Palareti G. Pharmacology and management of the vitamin K antagonists: American College of Chest Physicians Evidence-Based Clinical Practice Guidelines (8th Edition). Chest. 2008;133(6 Suppl):160S–98.

40. Dentali F, Ageno W, Crowther M. Treatment of coumarin-associated coagulopathy: a systematic review and proposed treatment algorithms. J Thromb Haemost. 2006;4(9):1853–63.

41. Crowther MA, Ageno W, Garcia D, Wang L, Witt DM, Clark NP, Blostein MD, Kahn SR, Vesely S, Schulman S, Kovacs MJ, Rodger

MA, Wells P, Anderson D, Ginsberg JS, Selby R, Siragusa S, Silingardi M, Dowd MB, Kearon C. Oral vitamin K versus placebo to correct excessive anticoagulation in patients receiving warfarin. Ann Intern Med. 2009;150:293–300.

42. Crowther MA, Douketis JD, Schnurr T, Steidl L, Mera V, Ultori C, Venco A, Ageno W. Oral vitamin K lowers the international normalized ratio more rapidly than subcutaneous vitamin K in the treatment of warfarin-associated coagulopathy. A randomized, controlled trial. Ann Intern Med. 2002;137(4):251–4.

43. Lubetsky A, Yonath H, Olchovsky D, Loebstein R, Halkin H, Ezra D. Comparison of oral vs intravenous phytonadione (vitamin K1) in patients with excessive anticoagulation: a prospective randomized controlled study. Arch Intern Med. 2003;163(20):2469–73.

44. Dentali F, Ageno W. Management of coumarin-associated coagulopathy in the non-bleeding patient: a systematic review. Haematologica. 2004;89(7):857–62.

45. Aguilar MI, Hart RG, Kase CS, Freeman WD, Hoeben BJ, Garcia RC, Ansell JE, Mayer SA, Norrving B, Rosand J, Steiner T, Wijdicks EF, Yamaguchi T, Yasaka M. Treatment of warfarin-associated intracerebral hemorrhage: literature review and expert opinion. Mayo Clin Proc. 2007;82(1):82–92.

46. van Aart L, Eijkhout HW, Kamphuis JS, Dam M, Schattenkerk ME, Schouten TJ, Ploeger B, Strengers PF. Individualized dosing regimen for prothrombin complex concentrate more effective than standard treatment in the reversal of oral anticoagulant therapy: an open, prospective randomized controlled trial. Thromb Res. 2006;118(3): 313–20.

47. Pabinger I, Brenner B, Kalina U, Knaub S, Nagy A, Ostermann H. Prothrombin complex concentrate (Beriplex P/N) for emergency anticoagulation reversal: a prospective multinational clinical trial. J Thromb Haemost. 2008;6(4):622–31.

48. Levi M. Disseminated intravascular coagulation. Crit Care Med. 2007;35:2191–5.

49. Levi M. New antithrombotics in the treatment of thromboembolic disease. Eur J Intern Med. 2005;16(4):230–7.

50. Strebel N, Prins M, Agnelli G, Buller HR. Preoperative or postoperative start of prophylaxis for venous thromboembolism with low-molecular-weight heparin in elective hip surgery? Arch Intern Med. 2002;162(13):1451–6.

51. Agnelli G, Gallus A, Goldhaber SZ, Haas S, Huisman MV, Hull RD, Kakkar AK, Misselwitz F, Schellong S. Treatment of proximal deep-vein thrombosis with the oral direct factor Xa inhibitor rivaroxaban (BAY 59–7939): the ODIXa-DVT (Oral Direct Factor Xa Inhibitor BAY 59–7939 in Patients With Acute Symptomatic Deep-Vein Thrombosis) study. Circulation. 2007;116(2):180–7.

52. Shantsila E, Lip GY. Apixaban, an oral, direct inhibitor of activated Factor Xa. Curr Opin Investig Drugs. 2008;9(9):1020–33.
53. Bauersachs R, Berkowitz SD, Brenner B, Buller HR, Decousus H, Gallus AS, Lensing AW, Misselwitz F, Prins MH, Raskob GE, Segers A, Verhamme P, Wells P, Agnelli G, Bounameaux H, Cohen A, Davidson BL, Piovella F, Schellong S. Oral rivaroxaban for symptomatic venous thromboembolism. N Engl J Med. 2010;363(26): 2499–510.
54. Buller HR, Prins MH, Lensin AW, Decousus H, Jacobson BF, Minar E, Chlumsky J, Verhamme P, Wells P, Agnelli G, Cohen A, Berkowitz SD, Bounameaux H, Davidson BL, Misselwitz F, Gallus AS, Raskob GE, Schellong S, Segers A. Oral rivaroxaban for the treatment of symptomatic pulmonary embolism. N Engl J Med. 2012;366(14): 1287–97.
55. Mega JL, Braunwald E, Mohanavelu S, Burton P, Poulter R, Misselwitz F, Hricak V, Barnathan ES, Bordes P, Witkowski A, Markov V, Oppenheimer L, Gibson CM. Rivaroxaban versus placebo in patients with acute coronary syndromes (ATLAS ACS-TIMI 46): a randomised, double-blind, phase II trial. Lancet. 2009; 374(9683):29–38.
56. Alexander JH, Becker RC, Bhatt DL, Cools F, Crea F, Dellborg M, Fox KA, Goodman SG, Harrington RA, Huber K, Husted S, Lewis BS, Lopez-Sendon J, Mohan P, Montalescot G, Ruda M, Ruzyllo W, Verheugt F, Wallentin L. Apixaban, an oral, direct, selective factor Xa inhibitor, in combination with antiplatelet therapy after acute coronary syndrome: results of the Apixaban for Prevention of Acute Ischemic and Safety Events (APPRAISE) trial. Circulation. 2009;119(22):2877–85.
57. Eerenberg ES, Kamphuisen PW, Sijpkens MK, Meijers JC, Buller HR, Levi M. Reversal of rivaroxaban and dabigatran by prothrombin complex concentrate: a randomized, placebo-controlled, crossover study in healthy subjects. Circulation. 2011;124:1573–9.
58. Fukuda T, Honda Y, Kamisato C, Morishima Y, Shibano T. Reversal of anticoagulant effects of edoxaban, an oral, direct factor Xa inhibitor, with haemostatic agents. Thromb Haemost. 2012;107(2):253–9.
59. Zhou W, Zorn M, Nawroth P, Butehorn U, Perzborn E, Heitmeier S, Veltkamp R. Hemostatic therapy in experimental intracerebral hemorrhage associated with rivaroxaban. Stroke. 2013;44(3): 771–8.
60. Marlu R, Hodaj E, Paris A, Albaladejo P, Cracowski JL, Pernod G. Effect of non-specific reversal agents on anticoagulant activity of dabigatran and rivaroxaban: a randomised crossover ex vivo study in healthy volunteers. Thromb Haemost. 2012;108(2):217–24.
61. Weitz JI, Buller HR. Direct thrombin inhibitors in acute coronary syndromes: present and future. Circulation. 2002;105(8):1004–11.

62. Wahlander K, Lapidus L, Olsson CG, Thuresson A, Eriksson UG, Larson G, Eriksson H. Pharmacokinetics, pharmacodynamics and clinical effects of the oral direct thrombin inhibitor ximelagatran in acute treatment of patients with pulmonary embolism and deep vein thrombosis. Thromb Res. 2002;107(3–4):93–9.

63. Eriksson BI, Smith H, Yasothan U, Kirkpatrick P. Dabigatran etexilate. Nat Rev Drug Discov. 2008;7(7):557–8.

64. Eriksson BI, Dahl OE, Rosencher N, Kurth AA, van Dijk CN, Frostick SP, Prins MH, Hettiarachchi R, Hantel S, Schnee J, Buller HR. Dabigatran etexilate versus enoxaparin for prevention of venous thromboembolism after total hip replacement: a randomised, double-blind, non-inferiority trial. Lancet. 2007;370(9591):949–56.

65. Connolly SJ, Ezekowitz MD, Yusuf S, Eikelboom J, Oldgren J, Parekh A, Pogue J, Reilly PA, Themeles E, Varrone J, Wang S, Alings M, Xavier D, Zhu J, Diaz R, Lewis BS, Darius H, Diener HC, Joyner CD, Wallentin L. Dabigatran versus warfarin in patients with atrial fibrillation. N Engl J Med. 2009;361(12):1139–51.

66. Woltz M, Levi M, Sarich TC, Bostrom SL, Erickson UG, Erikkson M, Svensson M, Weitz JI, Elg M, Wahlander K. Effect of recombinant factor VIIa on melagatran-induced inhibition of thrombin generation and platelet activation in healthy volunteers. Thromb Haemost. 2004;91:1090–6.

67. Zhou W, Schwarting S, Illanes S, Liesz A, Middelhoff M, Zorn M, Bendszus M, Heiland S, Van RJ, Veltkamp R. Hemostatic therapy in experimental intracerebral hemorrhage associated with the direct thrombin inhibitor dabigatran. Stroke. 2011;42(12):3594–9.

68. Patrono C, Baigent C, Hirsh J, Roth G. Antiplatelet drugs: American College of Chest Physicians Evidence-Based Clinical Practice Guidelines (8th Edition). Chest. 2008;133(6 Suppl):199S–233.

69. Merritt JC, Bhatt DL. The efficacy and safety of perioperative antiplatelet therapy. J Thromb Thrombolysis. 2004;17(1):21–7.

70. Richardson DW, Robinson AG. Desmopressin. [Review] [165 refs]. Ann Intern Med. 1985;103(2):228–39.

71. Reiter RA, Mayr F, Blazicek H, Galehr E, Jilma-Stohlawetz P, Domanovits H, Jilma B. Desmopressin antagonizes the in vitro platelet dysfunction induced by GPIIb/IIIa inhibitors and aspirin. Blood. 2003;102(13):4594–9.

72. Anonymous. A randomised, blinded, trial of clopidogrel versus aspirin in patients at risk of ischaemic events (CAPRIE). CAPRIE Steering Committee [see comments]. Lancet. 1996;348(9038):1329–39.

73. Yusuf S, Zhao F, Mehta SR, Chrolavicius S, Tognoni G, Fox KK. Effects of clopidogrel in addition to aspirin in patients with acute coronary syndromes without ST-segment elevation. N Engl J Med. 2001;345(7):494–502.

74. Bhatt DL. Prasugrel in clinical practice. N Engl J Med. 2009;361(10):940–2.

75. Montalescot G, Wiviott SD, Braunwald E, Murphy SA, Gibson CM, McCabe CH, Antman EM. Prasugrel compared with clopidogrel in patients undergoing percutaneous coronary intervention for ST-elevation myocardial infarction (TRITON-TIMI 38): double-blind, randomised controlled trial. Lancet. 2009;373(9665):723–31.

76. Wiviott SD, Braunwald E, McCabe CH, Montalescot G, Ruzyllo W, Gottlieb S, Neumann FJ, Ardissino D, De SS, Murphy SA, Riesmeyer J, Weerakkody G, Gibson CM, Antman EM. Prasugrel versus clopidogrel in patients with acute coronary syndromes. N Engl J Med. 2007;357(20):2001–15.

77. Giannitsis E, Katus A. Antiplatelet therapy – ticagrelor. Hamostaseologie. 2012;32:177–85.

78. Wallentin L, Becker RC, Budaj A, Cannon CP, Emanuelsson H, Held C, et al. Ticagrelor versus clopidogrel in patients with acute coronary syndromes. N Engl J Med. 2009;361:1045–57.

79. Bhatt DL, Lincoff AM, Gibson CM, Stone GW, McNulty S, Montalescot G, Kleiman NS, Goodman SG, White HD, Mahaffey KW, Pollack Jr CV, Manoukian SV, Widimsky P, Chew DP, Cura F, Manukov I, Tousek F, Jafar MZ, Arneja J, Skerjanec S, Harrington RA. Intravenous platelet blockade with cangrelor during PCI. N Engl J Med. 2009;361(24):2330–41.

80. Harrington RA, Stone GW, McNulty S, White HD, Lincoff AM, Gibson CM, Pollack Jr CV, Montalescot G, Mahaffey KW, Kleiman NS, Goodman SG, Amine M, Angiolillo DJ, Becker RC, Chew DP, French WJ, Leisch F, Parikh KH, Skerjanec S, Bhatt DL. Platelet inhibition with cangrelor in patients undergoing PCI. N Engl J Med. 2009;361(24):2318–29.

81. Grines CL, Bonow RO, Casey Jr DE, Gardner TJ, Lockhart PB, Moliterno DJ, O'Gara P, Whitlow P. Prevention of premature discontinuation of dual antiplatelet therapy in patients with coronary artery stents: a science advisory from the American Heart Association, American College of Cardiology, Society for Cardiovascular Angiography and Interventions, American College of Surgeons, and American Dental Association, with representation from the American College of Physicians. Catheter Cardiovasc Interv. 2007;69(3):334–40.

82. Vilahur G, Choi BG, Zafar MU, Viles-Gonzalez JF, Vorchheimer DA, Fuster V, Badimon JJ. Normalization of platelet reactivity in clopidogrel-treated subjects. J Thromb Haemost. 2007;5(1):82–90.

83. Leithauser B, Zielske D, Seyfert UT, Jung F. Effects of desmopressin on platelet membrane glycoproteins and platelet aggregation in volunteers on clopidogrel. Clin Hemorheol Microcirc. 2008;39(1–4): 293–302.

Index

P. Avanzas, P. Clemmensen (eds.), *Pharmacological Treatment*   239
of Acute Coronary Syndromes, Current Cardiovascular Therapy,
DOI 10.1007/978-1-4471-5424-2,
© Springer-Verlag London 2014

240   Index

9781447154235